# ULTIMATE
## GUIDE TO GOLF
### THE JOURNEY BEGINS

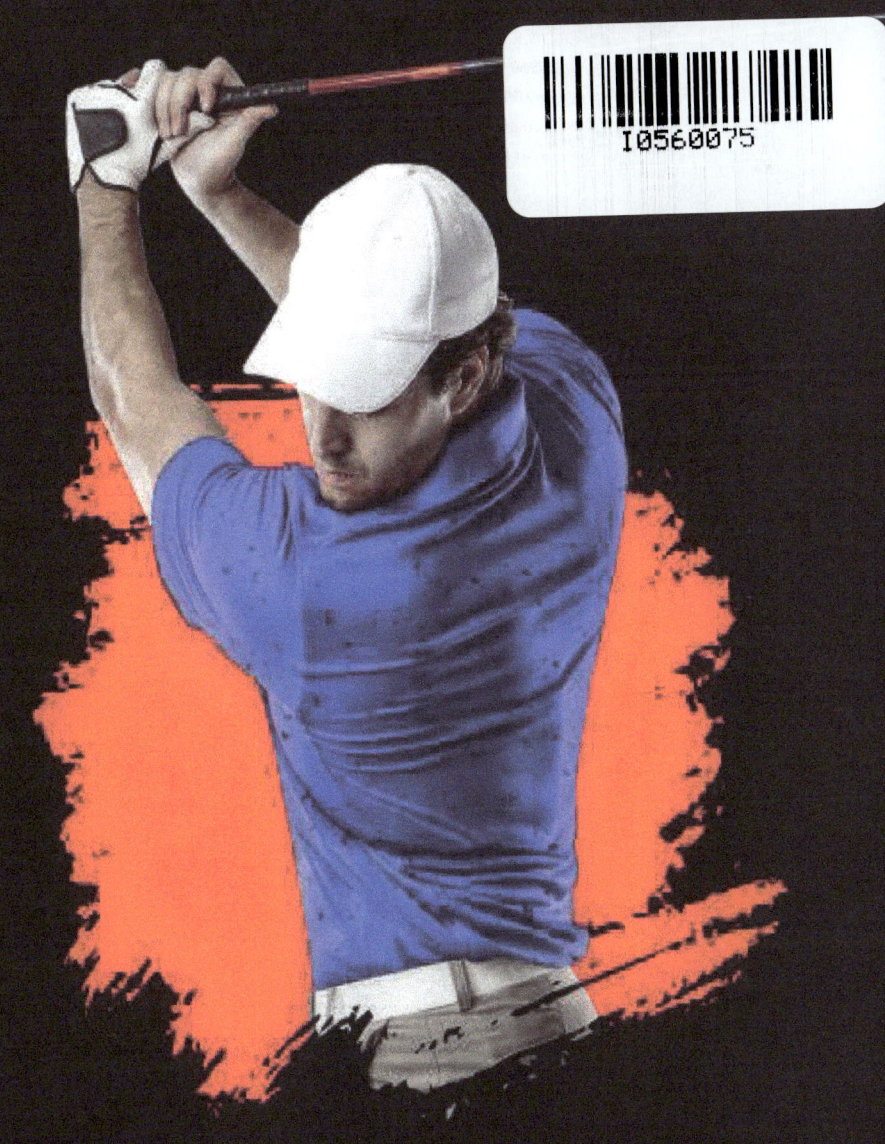

# ULTIMATE GUIDE TO GOLF

# THE JOURNEY BEGINS

DEDICATED TO MY GOLF STUDENTS
PAST, CURRENT, AND FUTURE
by
Glen Bowen

Certified Professional Golf Coach
United States Golf Teachers Federation

Champion Club Member
United States Golf Association

*Additional Golf Books by Glen Bowen*

*Scoring Magic – Transform Your Short Game Today*
*Golf Decoded – Beginner's Guide*
*Mind Over Mulligan – Mastering Your Mindset*
*Golden Greens – Golfing Through Life's Back Nine*
*Optimization of the Golf Swing – Biomechanics*
*Junior Golfers – The Parents Guidebook*

*Golfopedia Trilogy – Golf Deconstructed*

*Front Nine – Mastering Golf from Ace to Zip*
*Back Nine – Exploring the Science Behind Golf*
*Nineteenth Hole – Wrapping Up Your Final Round*

# Introduction

Golf transcends time, culture, and skill. It challenges both body and mind with precision, patience, and perseverance. Whether stepping onto the course for the first time or refining your swing after years of practice, golf is a journey of self-discovery and growth. Its universal appeal makes it more than a pastime—it's a lifelong pursuit.

The origins of golf date back centuries, with its modern form emerging in 15th-century Scotland. From these beginnings to today's global sport, golf has evolved into a beloved pastime for millions. Its history is rich in tradition yet embraces innovations in technology and technique, blending heritage with modernity.

For those new to golf, this book is your guide. Golf may seem daunting—rules, equipment, etiquette—but every golfer starts somewhere. This guide simplifies the basics, building confidence as you step onto the fairway. From gripping a club to navigating a course, it provides all you need to begin.

Additionally, experienced players will benefit from new insights herein and refreshed memories long forgotten. Golf is a game of constant growth. This guide explores new swing techniques, strategies to improve your game, and advice on choosing equipment suited for your game. Whether aiming for consistency or perfection, this book can elevate your performance.

*Ultimate Guide to Golf* is more than an instructional book; it's an invitation into golf culture. It spans the sport's history, modern equipment innovations, and swing analysis. You'll learn how to play and why so many are captivated by this game.

As you turn these pages, remember that golf is more than hitting a ball—it's about embracing challenges and joy in beautiful open spaces. Whether learning or improving, this book will guide your every step.

Welcome to the wonderful world of golf!

# Contents

# Introduction to Golf

## Origins of Golf

The origins of golf can be traced back to Scotland in the mid-15th century, though similar stick-and-ball games existed earlier in history. Evidence suggests that golf-like games were played in China during the Song Dynasty (960–1279) and in the Netherlands, where players used sticks to hit leather balls toward a target. However, modern golf as we know it originated in Scotland, where its defining feature—the hole—was introduced. The first official mention of golf occurred in 1457 when King James II of Scotland banned it because he believed it distracted from military training, particularly archery practice. This ban was lifted in 1502 with the Treaty of Glasgow when King James IV became an avid golfer himself.

## Evolution into the Modern Game

Golf began evolving into its modern form during the 16th century when its popularity spread across Europe due to royal influence. Mary Queen of Scots introduced the game to France while studying there, and King Charles I brought it to England. By 1744, formal rules for golf were established by the Honourable Company of Edinburgh Golfers, who published a set of 13 articles known as "Articles and Laws in Playing at Golf." These rules were later adopted by the Royal and Ancient Golf Club of St Andrews (founded in 1754), which became one of the sport's governing bodies.

The construction of an 18-hole course at St Andrews in 1764 set the standard for modern golf courses. During this period, equipment also evolved: wooden clubs made from beech or ash and feather-filled balls gave way to more advanced materials over time.

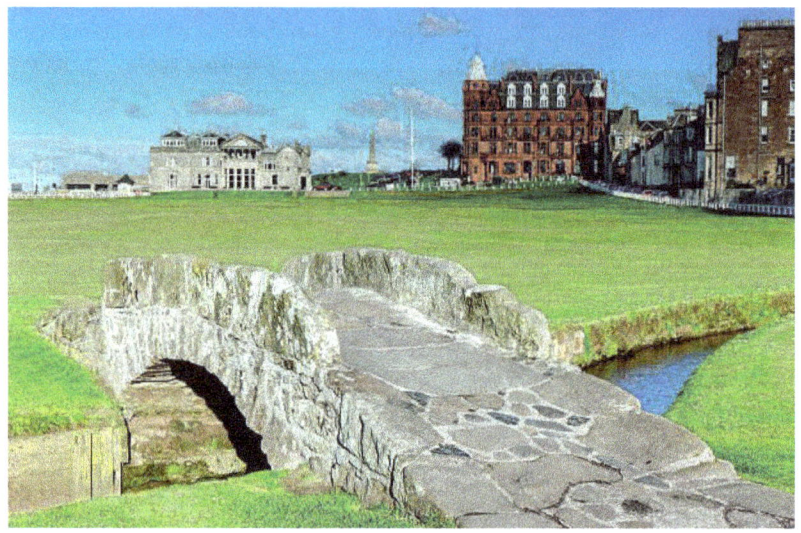

In the 19th century, golf expanded globally through Scottish expatriates and British colonial influence. The Industrial Revolution made travel easier via railways and enabled mass production of equipment, making golf accessible to more people. Prestwick Golf Club hosted the first British Open Championship in 1860, marking a significant milestone for competitive play.

Golf reached America by the late 18th century but gained traction only after the establishment of clubs like St Andrew's Golf Club (New York) in 1888 and organizations such as the United States Golf Association (USGA) in 1894. By 1900, over a thousand clubs had formed across America. The introduction of commercial sponsorships further professionalized the sport.

Today, golf is played worldwide on diverse courses ranging from manicured parklands in America to rugged links courses in Britain.

Iconic tournaments like The Masters and The Open Championship continue to celebrate its rich history while showcasing its evolution into a global phenomenon.

The Journey Begins

# Why Play Golf

Golf is a unique sport that offers a wide range of benefits, encompassing physical fitness, mental focus, social interaction, and the development of life skills such as patience and perseverance. Below is a detailed breakdown of these benefits:

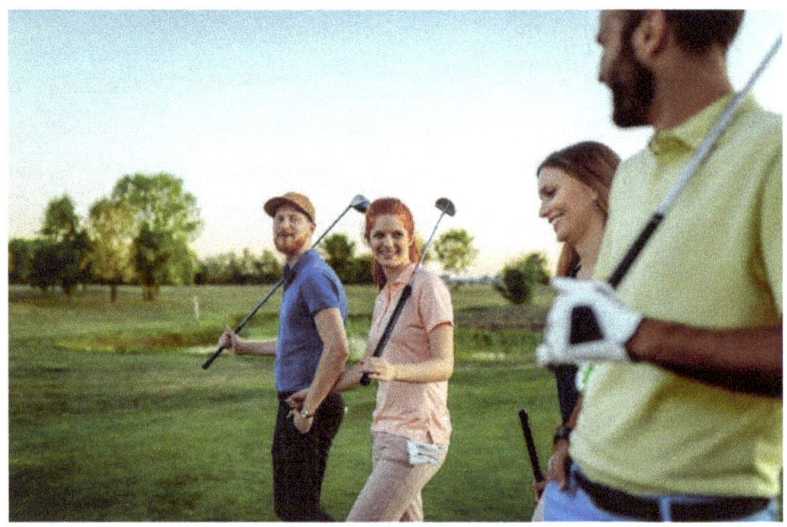

## Physical Fitness

Playing golf provides numerous physical health benefits, making it an excellent choice for individuals looking to stay active. A typical round of golf involves walking an average of 5 to 7 kilometers (3 to 4 miles) on an 18-hole course. This level of activity contributes significantly to cardiovascular health by improving endurance and promoting heart health. Walking regularly during golf helps burn calories—approximately 300-500 calories per hour depending on factors like terrain and whether you carry or pull your clubs.

Additionally, swinging a golf club engages multiple muscle groups, including those in the arms, shoulders, back, and core. Over time, this repetitive motion can improve muscle tone and strength while enhancing flexibility. Carrying or pulling your own clubs further increases calorie expenditure and builds stamina.

Golf also supports weight management by reducing body fat when played consistently. The low-impact nature of the sport makes it accessible to people of all ages and fitness levels while minimizing the risk of injury compared to high-impact sports.

## Mental Focus

Golf is not just a physical game but also a mental challenge that sharpens focus and concentration. Each shot requires careful planning, precision, and decision-making as players assess factors like wind direction, terrain conditions, and distance to the hole. This process fosters problem-solving skills and encourages creative thinking.

The sport also promotes mindfulness by requiring players to remain present in the moment. Concentrating on each swing or putt helps reduce distractions from everyday stressors. Furthermore, being outdoors in natural surroundings has been shown to lower anxiety levels and improve overall mental well-being.

Golf's emphasis on strategy enhances cognitive functions such as memory retention (e.g., recalling yardages or previous shots) and spatial awareness (e.g., visualizing ball trajectories). These mental exercises contribute to long-term brain health by keeping the mind active.

## Social Interaction

Golf is inherently social, offering opportunities for meaningful connections with others while fostering camaraderie among players. Whether playing with friends, family members, or new acquaintances at a local course or club event, golf creates an environment conducive to conversation and bonding.

The relaxed pace of the game allows for extended interactions between shots without feeling rushed—a rarity in many other sports. Socializing during golf can boost self-esteem and combat feelings of loneliness or isolation.

For beginners or those looking to expand their network, joining group lessons, or participating in tournaments provides opportunities to meet new people who share similar interests. The shared experience of navigating challenges on the course often leads to lasting friendships.

## Life Skills: Patience & Perseverance

Golf teaches valuable life skills such as patience, perseverance, discipline, and emotional resilience. The game's inherent difficulty requires players to accept setbacks gracefully—whether it's missing a putt or landing in a bunker—and motivates them to keep improving through practice.

Patience is cultivated as players learn that progress takes time; mastering techniques like driving accuracy or putting consistency doesn't happen overnight. Golf also reinforces perseverance by encouraging individuals to overcome obstacles (both literal hazards on the course and figurative challenges like frustration).

Discipline plays a key role in maintaining proper form during swings or adhering to rules governing fair play. Additionally, managing emotions after poor shots fosters emotional control—a skill transferable beyond sports into everyday life situations.

Finally, setting personal goals (e.g., lowering one's handicap) instills motivation while providing measurable benchmarks for success over time.

## Additional Benefits

- Connection with Nature: Playing golf often takes place in scenic environments filled with greenery and fresh air. Spending time outdoors has been linked to improved mood and reduced stress.

- Vitamin D Exposure: Being outside under sunlight helps maintain healthy vitamin D levels essential for bone health and immune function.

- Low Injury Risk: Golf is considered a low-impact sport compared to activities like running or contact sports; this makes it suitable for older adults or those recovering from injuries.

- Flexibility & Balance: Regular play improves joint mobility while enhancing balance through controlled movements during swings.

# The Journey Counts More

Golf is a sport that offers a lifetime of enjoyment, challenge, and personal growth. Whether you're just starting out or playing casually on weekends, it's important to approach the game with patience, realistic expectations, and a willingness to learn. This final chapter will summarize key takeaways for beginner golfers and weekend players while offering practical advice to help you continue improving and enjoying the game.

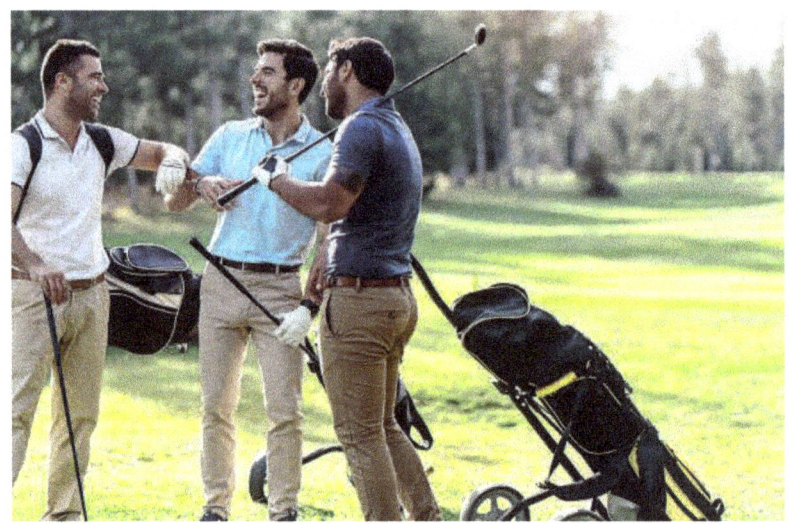

## 1. Embrace the Journey

Golf is not a sport that can be mastered overnight. It requires time, effort, and persistence. As a beginner or casual player, focus on progress rather than perfection. Celebrate small victories like hitting your first straight drive, making consistent contact with the ball, or completing an entire round without losing too many balls.

- **Set Realistic Goals:** Instead of aiming to shoot par right away, set achievable goals like breaking 100 or simply improving your short game.

- **Enjoy the Process:** Remember that every golfer—no matter their skill level—has bad days on the course. Learn from mistakes and keep moving forward.

- **Stay Patient:** Improvement in golf often comes in small increments. Trust that consistent practice will lead to better results over time.

## 2. Build a Solid Foundation

As a beginner golfer, or as a high handicapper, your primary focus should be on developing fundamental skills and understanding the basics of the game.

- **Master the Basics:** Spend time learning proper grip, stance, posture, and alignment. These fundamentals are critical for building a repeatable swing.

- **Practice Smartly:** Instead of mindlessly hitting balls at the driving range, work on specific aspects of your game such as chipping around the green or putting accuracy.

- **Learn Course Etiquette:** Understanding golf etiquette—like repairing divots, raking bunkers, and keeping pace—is just as important as learning how to swing a club.

## 3. Invest in Beginner-Friendly Equipment

You don't need expensive clubs or high-end gear when starting out. A basic set of beginner-friendly clubs will suffice until you develop more consistency in your swing.

- Look for affordable sets with forgiving club designs (e.g., cavity-back irons) that make it easier to hit good shots.

- Consider renting clubs if you're unsure about committing to buying your own set right away.

- Don't forget essential accessories like golf balls (choose budget-friendly ones), tees, gloves, and comfortable shoes.

## 4. Focus on Short Game Mastery

While it's tempting to spend all your practice time trying to hit long drives at the range, most strokes in golf are made within 100 yards of the hole. Improving your short game can significantly lower your scores.

- Practice putting regularly: Work on distance control (lag putting) and short putts inside 5 feet.

- Hone your chipping skills: Learn how to use wedges effectively around greens.

- Experiment with bunker shots: Practice getting out of sand traps smoothly, so they don't intimidate you during rounds.

## 5. Play Strategically

Golf isn't just about hitting great shots; it's also about managing your way around the course intelligently.

- Play within Your Limits: Avoid risky shots that could lead to penalties or lost balls.

- Choose Appropriate Tees: Play from tees that match your skill level so you can enjoy the round without feeling overwhelmed by long distances.

- Develop Course Awareness: Pay attention to hazards like bunkers and water features when planning each shot.

## 6. Make Golf Fun

At its core, golf is meant to be an enjoyable experience—especially for weekend players who use it as a way to relax and unwind.

- Play with Friends: Golf is more fun when shared with others! Invite friends or join local leagues for social rounds.

- Explore New Courses: Challenge yourself by playing different courses in your area or during vacations.

- Keep Perspective: Don't let bad shots ruin your day; remember why you started playing in the first place—to have fun.

## 7. Continue Learning

Even as a casual golfer, there's always room for improvement—and plenty of resources available to help you grow as a player.

- Watch Instructional Videos: Platforms like YouTube offer free tutorials covering everything from swing mechanics to mental strategies.

- Take Lessons: Consider investing in lessons with a PGA professional who can provide personalized feedback tailored specifically for you.

- Read Books/Articles: Dive into books written by experienced golfers or browse online guides tailored toward beginners looking for tips on technique and strategy.

## 8. Stay Physically Active

Golf may not seem as physically demanding as other sports but maintaining good fitness levels can improve both performance and enjoyment on the course.

- Stretch Regularly: Flexibility is key for executing smooth swings without risking injury.

- Build Core Strength: A strong core helps generate power while maintaining balance throughout swings.

- Walk When Possible: Opting not to use carts adds extra exercise value during rounds while allowing more connection with nature.

## 9. Celebrate Progress

Finally—and perhaps most importantly—take time after each round or practice session to reflect on what went well rather than dwelling solely on mistakes made along the way!

Celebrate milestones big (breaking 90!) AND small (hitting fewer slices). By focusing positively instead negatively—you'll stay motivated continue striving toward becoming better golfer overall!

# Basic Overview:
# How to Play a Hole

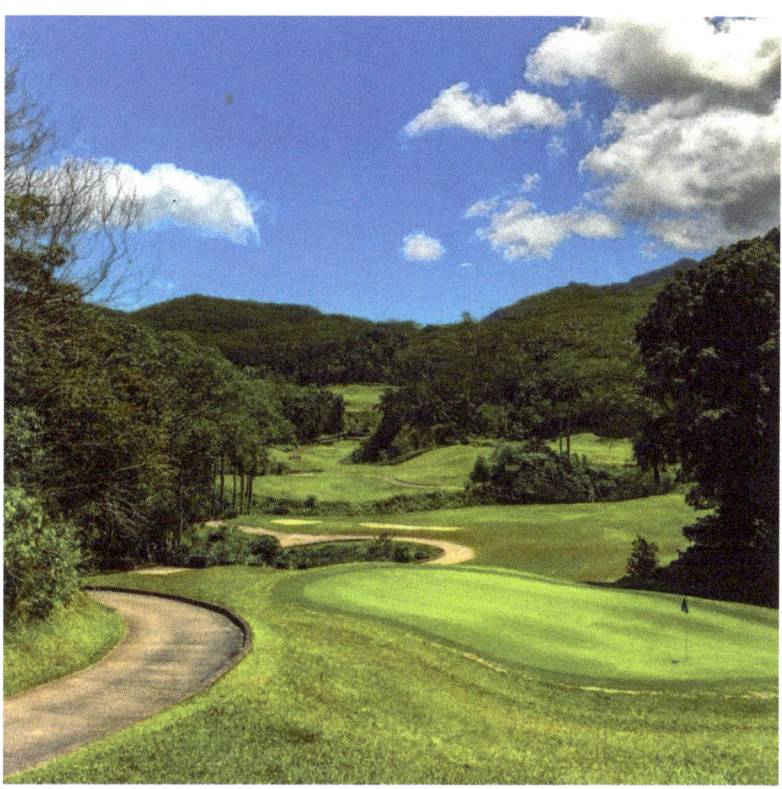

Golf is played on a course that consists of a series of holes, typically 18, though some courses may have 9. Each hole begins at the teeing area, where players take their first shot (called the "tee shot") using a club of their choice. The goal is to hit the ball into the hole located on the green (a closely mowed area) in as few strokes as possible. Players progress from where their ball lands after each stroke until they successfully sink it into the hole.

Each hole has a designated par, which represents the number of strokes an expert golfer is expected to need to complete that hole. Par includes two putts, assuming the golfer reaches the green in regulation (the expected number of strokes to reach the green). Holes are classified by par values: par-3, par-4, or par-5, depending on their length and difficulty.

## Scoring Basics: Understanding Par and Common Terms

### Par

Par is the baseline score for each hole. For example:

- o   A par-3 hole expects completion in 3 strokes.

- o   A par-4 hole expects completion in 4 strokes.

- o   A par-5 hole expects completion in 5 strokes.

### Birdie

A birdie occurs when a player completes a hole in one stroke under par. For instance:

- o   Scoring 2 on a par-3.

- o   Scoring 3 on a par-4.

- o   Scoring 4 on a par-5.

### Bogey

A bogey happens when a player takes one stroke over par to finish a hole. For example:

- o   Scoring 4 on a par-3.

- ○ Scoring 5 on a par-4.

- ○ Scoring 6 on a par-5.

## Eagle

An eagle is achieved when completing a hole in two strokes under par, such as:

- ○ Scoring 1 (a hole-in-one) on a par-3.

- ○ Scoring 2 on a par-4.

- ○ Scoring 3 on a par-5.

## Double Bogey and Beyond

A double bogey means finishing the hole in two strokes over par, while higher scores are referred to with additional prefixes (e.g., triple bogey for three over, quadruple bogey for four over).

## Hole-in-One (Ace)

This rare achievement occurs when the ball is sunk with just one stroke from the teeing area, regardless of the hole's designated par.

# Key Rules for Playing Golf

## Order of Play:

The player farthest from the hole plays first after tee shots, ensuring fairness and safety during play.

## Tee Shots:

Players must begin each hole by hitting their ball from within or behind the designated tee markers without crossing them.

**Ball Placement:**

After every shot, players must play their next shot from where their ball comes to rest unless specific rules allow otherwise (e.g., penalties or relief situations).

**Penalty Strokes:**

Penalty strokes are added for rule violations such as hitting out-of-bounds, losing your ball, or taking an unplayable lie.

**Putting:**

On reaching the green, players use putters to roll their balls into the cup while avoiding interference with other players' lines of play.

**Etiquette:**

Golf emphasizes respect for others and maintaining pace of play by not delaying unnecessarily between shots.

# Equipment Basics

## Golf Clubs

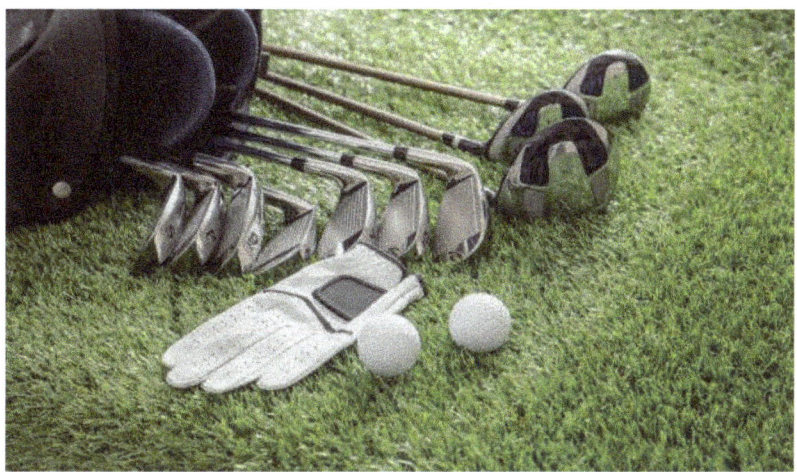

Golf clubs are essential tools in the game of golf, and each type of club is designed for specific purposes to help players navigate different situations on the course. A standard set of golf clubs typically includes a combination of drivers, irons, wedges, hybrids, and putters. Below is a detailed explanation of the main types of clubs and their uses:

### Driver

The driver, also known as the 1-wood, is the longest club in a golfer's bag and is primarily used for hitting long-distance shots off the tee.

- Design: Drivers have large, hollow clubheads with low loft angles (typically between 7 and 12 degrees) to maximize distance. The shaft is also the longest among all clubs, which allows for faster swing speeds.

- Purpose: The driver is used to achieve maximum distance on par-4 or par-5 holes where golfers need to cover significant yardage from the tee box.

- Modern Trends: In recent years, professional golfers have shifted toward higher-lofted drivers (10–11 degrees) to achieve an optimal combination of high launch angles and low spin rates for longer drives.

**Irons**

Irons are versatile clubs that come in numbered sets (e.g., 3-iron through 9-iron) and are used for a variety of shots depending on their loft.

- Design: Irons have smaller clubheads compared to woods, with angled faces (lofts) that impart spin on the ball. They can be solid or hollow-headed. As the number increases (e.g., from 3 to 9), the loft increases while shaft length decreases.

- Purpose:
  - Lower-numbered irons (3–5): Used for longer approach shots or when hitting from fairways or roughs at distances typically ranging from 150–200 yards.
  - Mid-irons (6–7): Used for moderate distances around 130–160 yards.
  - Higher-numbered irons (8–9): Designed for shorter approach shots into greens or precision shots requiring more control.

- Usage: Irons are commonly used on fairways but can also be employed for tee shots on shorter holes.

## Wedges

Wedges are specialized irons with higher lofts designed for short-distance precision shots around greens or out of challenging lies like sand bunkers.

- Types of Wedges:

  o Pitching Wedge (PW): Typically has a loft between 44–48 degrees and is used for approach shots from about 100–130 yards.

  o Gap Wedge (GW): Fills the gap between pitching and sand wedges with a loft around 50–54 degrees; ideal for controlled approach shots.

  o Sand Wedge (SW): With a loft between 54–58 degrees, it's specifically designed to help golfers escape sand bunkers or hit high-lofted chips around greens.

  o Lob Wedge (LW): The highest-lofted wedge (58–64 degrees), used for very short pitches or chips requiring height and stopping power near the hole.

- Purpose: Wedges provide accuracy and control in short-game scenarios where finesse is critical.

## Putter

The putter is one of the most important clubs in golf because it's used on the green to roll the ball into the hole.

- Design: Putters come in various shapes and sizes but generally feature flat faces with minimal loft (around 3–4 degrees). Common styles include:

- o Blade Putters: Traditional design with narrow heads; preferred by players who value precision over forgiveness.

- o Mallet Putters: Larger heads offering better stability and forgiveness on off-center hits.

- o Heel-Toe Weighted Putters: A hybrid design that balances forgiveness and precision.

**Additionally, putters vary in length:**

- o Standard-Length Putters: Range from about 32 to 36 inches; suitable for most players.

- o Belly Putters & Long Putters: Longer designs that allow anchoring against parts of the body like the belly or chest; these are less common due to rule changes restricting anchoring techniques during play.

- • Purpose: The putter is exclusively used on putting greens where accuracy rather than power determines success. Its goal is to start rolling the ball smoothly toward its target without excessive backspin or skidding.

## Summary

Each type of golf club serves a unique purpose based on its design characteristics such as loft angle, shaft length, head size, and weight distribution. Drivers excel at long-distance tee shots; irons provide versatility across varying distances; wedges specialize in short-game finesse; and putters are indispensable tools for finishing holes effectively.

# Golf Balls

Modern golf balls are highly engineered products made up of multiple components that work together to optimize performance for different types of golfers. Here's how they are designed:

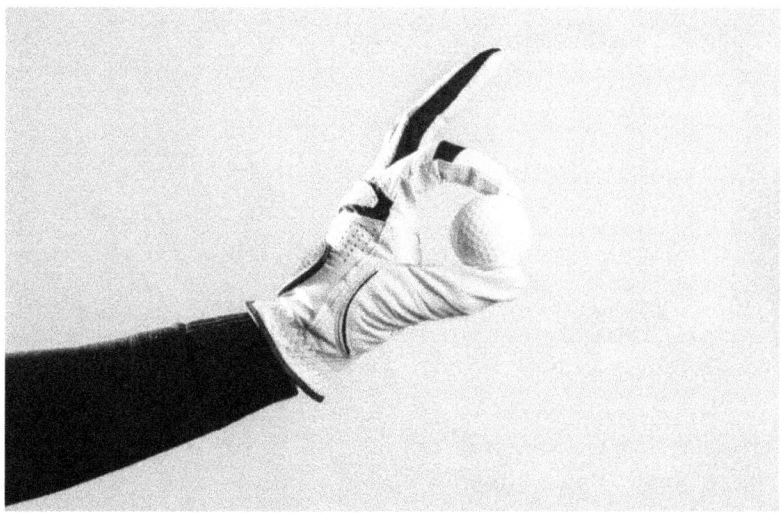

## Core

The core is often referred to as the "engine" of the golf ball because it plays a central role in determining speed, distance, and spin. It is typically made from pressurized rubber or synthetic materials that store and release energy upon impact with the clubface.

- **High-compression cores** (harder cores) generate more energy transfer for faster swing speeds, resulting in greater distance.

- **Low-compression cores** (softer cores) compress more easily on impact, making them ideal for slower swing speeds as they help maximize distance without requiring excessive force.

Some advanced multi-layer balls include dual or multi-material cores to fine-tune performance characteristics like spin control or launch angle.

## Mantle Layers

In multi-layer golf balls, mantle layers sit between the core and the outer cover. These layers are designed to influence spin rates and energy transfer:

- They reduce driver spin for longer shots off the tee.

- They increase wedge spin for better control around greens. Mantle layers also help balance compression differences between the core and cover.

## Cover

The outermost layer of a golf ball is its cover, which significantly affects feel, durability, and spin:

- **Urethane covers**: Found on premium balls; these provide excellent short-game spin and soft feel but are less durable.

- **Surlyn covers**: More durable but offer less spin control; common in mid-range or beginner-level balls. The cover also features dimples that play a crucial role in aerodynamics.

## Dimples

Dimples on a golf ball reduce air resistance (drag) while increasing lift by creating turbulence around the ball as it flies through the air. This allows it to travel farther with a stable trajectory. The number, size, depth, and pattern of dimples vary across models but typically range from 300 to 500 dimples per ball.

# Key Performance Factors Influenced by Design

## Distance

The combination of core compression, mantle layers, and dimple patterns determines how far a ball will travel when struck with maximum force. High-compression balls with optimized aerodynamics tend to deliver greater distances for players with faster swing speeds.

## Spin

Spin rates vary depending on shot type:

- Low-spin balls reduce sidespin off drivers to minimize slices or hooks.

- High-spin balls enhance backspin for better control during approach shots or chips around greens. Multi-layer designs allow manufacturers to fine-tune these characteristics based on player needs.

## Trajectory

Dimples not only affect distance but also influence trajectory by controlling lift forces acting on the ball during flight. Some models are designed for higher trajectories (ideal for stopping power on greens), while others promote lower trajectories (better in windy conditions).

## Feel

Feel refers to how soft or firm a ball feels when struck. This is largely determined by cover material and compression:

- Softer-feeling balls (low compression): Preferred by players who prioritize touch around greens.

- Firmer-feeling balls (high compression): Favored by those seeking maximum feedback on full swings.

# Why Golf Balls Matter

Golfers use their ball on every single shot during a round—making it arguably the most important piece of equipment in their bag. Here's why choosing the right one matters:

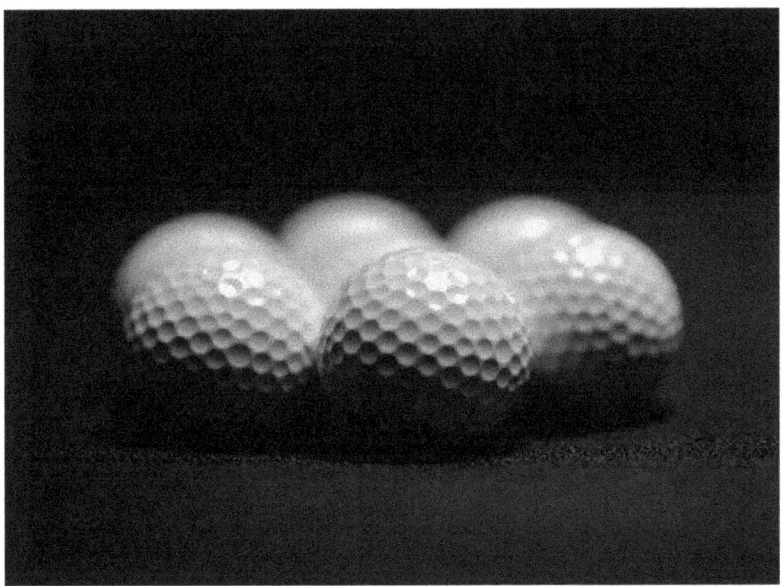

## Tailoring Performance to Skill Level

Different golfers have varying swing speeds, shot preferences, and skill levels:

- Beginners may benefit from two-piece construction balls with low compression for added forgiveness and distance.

- Advanced players often prefer multi-layer urethane-covered balls that offer precise control over spin rates.

## Maximizing Consistency

A well-suited golf ball ensures consistent results across all types of shots—from drives off the tee to delicate putts on the green—helping golfers improve their scores over time.

## Enhancing Confidence

Using a golf ball that aligns with your playing style can boost confidence during rounds. For example:

- A high-spin model might give skilled players more confidence attacking pins.

- A low-spin model could help beginners avoid errant shots like slices or hooks.

## Types of Golf Balls

There are three main categories based on construction:

**Two-Piece Balls:**

- o Simple design with a large core covered by Surlyn.

- o Prioritize durability and distance over feel or spin.

- o Ideal for beginners or casual players due to affordability.

**Three-Piece Balls:**

- o Add an intermediate layer between core and cover.

- o Offer better control than two-piece models while maintaining decent distance.

o   Suitable for intermediate golfers seeking balanced performance.

**Four-Piece (or Multi-Layered):**

o   Include multiple mantle layers plus urethane covers.

o   Deliver exceptional short-game control without sacrificing long-game performance.

o   Preferred by advanced players who demand versatility across all aspects of their game.

Golf balls are meticulously designed pieces of equipment that combine physics, engineering, and materials science to meet diverse player needs across all skill levels. Their construction—including core composition, mantle layers, cover material, dimple patterns—directly influences key factors like distance, spin rate, trajectory control, durability, and feel. Selecting the right golf ball tailored to your playing style can significantly enhance your overall performance on the course while building consistency in your game over time.

# Other Essential Items

## Tees

Tees are small objects used to elevate the golf ball off the ground for an easier shot, primarily on the first stroke of each hole. They are typically made from wood or plastic and come in various sizes to accommodate different club types and player preferences.

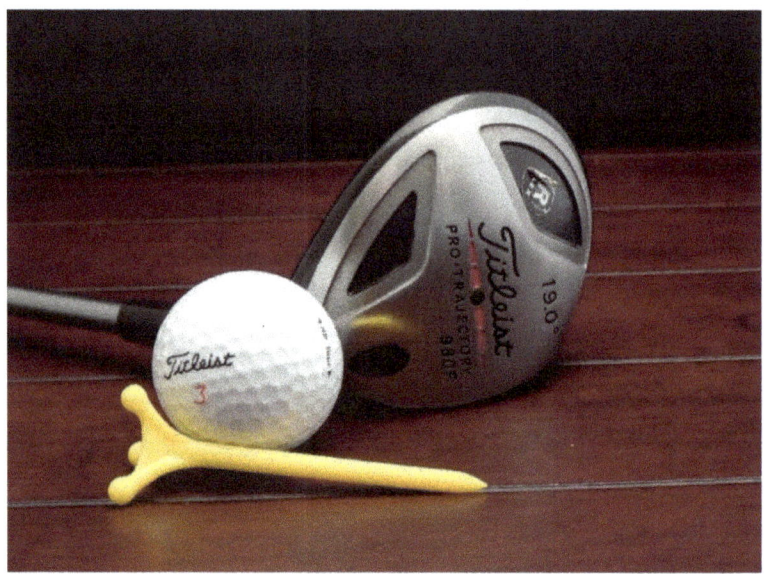

- Sizes: Tees range in height, with longer tees often preferred by beginners as they can be pushed further into the ground for stability. The height of the tee should complement your swing style and club choice (e.g., drivers require higher tees compared to irons).

- Material: Wooden tees are biodegradable but may break more easily, while plastic tees are more durable but less environmentally friendly.

- Selection Tips: Beginners should experiment with different tee heights to find what feels most comfortable during their opening shots. There is no need to invest in expensive or branded tees at this stage since performance differences are minimal.

## Gloves

Golf gloves are designed to improve grip, prevent blisters, and provide comfort during play. Most golfers wear a glove on their non-dominant hand (e.g., left hand for right-handed players).

- Purpose: Gloves enhance grip by reducing slippage caused by sweat or moisture. They also protect hands from developing calluses or blisters during repetitive swings.

- Fit: A properly fitting glove is crucial—it should feel snug without restricting movement or cutting off circulation. Loose gloves can compromise grip effectiveness.

- Material Options:
  - Leather gloves offer excellent grip and durability but can be more expensive.
  - Synthetic gloves are affordable and perform well in wet conditions but may wear out faster.
  - Hybrid gloves combine leather palms with synthetic backs for a balance of durability and flexibility.

- Care Tips: To extend the life of your glove, allow it to air dry after use and avoid storing it in damp conditions.

## Shoes with Spikes/Traction Soles

Golf shoes are essential for maintaining stability and comfort throughout a round of golf, especially given the varied terrain encountered on courses.

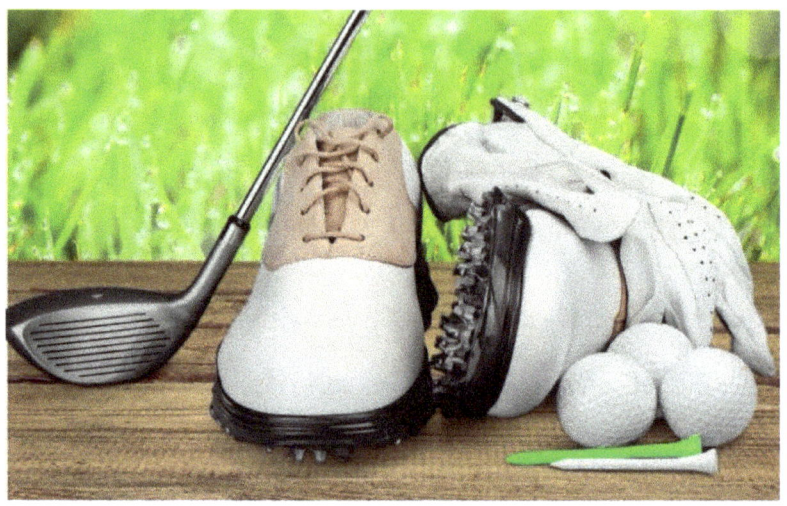

**Spiked Shoes:**

- These feature replaceable cleats on the soles that provide superior traction on grass, particularly in wet or uneven conditions.

- Modern spiked shoes often use soft plastic cleats instead of traditional metal spikes, which are gentler on greens while still offering excellent grip.

**Spikeless Shoes:**

- Spikeless designs have rubber nubs or patterns on the sole that provide traction without cleats. These shoes are versatile as they can be worn both on and off the course.

o While spikeless shoes may not offer as much grip as spiked ones in slippery conditions, they tend to be lighter and more comfortable for walking long distances.

**Key Features to Look For:**

o Water Resistance: Golfers often encounter dew-covered grass or rain; water-resistant shoes help keep feet dry.

o Comfort: Since golf involves significant walking (often several miles per round), cushioning and arch support are critical.

o Durability: High-quality materials ensure longevity despite exposure to rough terrain.

- Cost Considerations: Name-brand golf shoes typically start at around $100 but can go higher depending on features like waterproofing or advanced materials. Beginners should look for sales at sporting goods stores or online retailers to find quality options at lower prices.

## For beginners focusing on golf essentials

1. Use affordable wooden or plastic tees that match your preferred height for driving shots.

2. Invest in a well-fitting glove made from leather, synthetic material, or a hybrid combination based on your budget and needs.

3. Choose golf shoes with either spiked soles for maximum traction or spikeless designs for versatility—prioritizing comfort, water resistance, and durability.

When selecting golf equipment for beginners, it is essential to focus on gear that enhances learning, improves performance, and ensures comfort. Beginners often face challenges in mastering the game's techniques, so choosing age-appropriate and beginner-friendly equipment can make a significant difference. Ahead are detailed tips on how to select the right equipment step by step:

## Choosing Golf Clubs:
## Prioritize Forgiveness and Ease of Use

Golf clubs are the most critical part of any golfer's equipment. For beginners, forgiving clubs that help compensate for mishits are ideal.

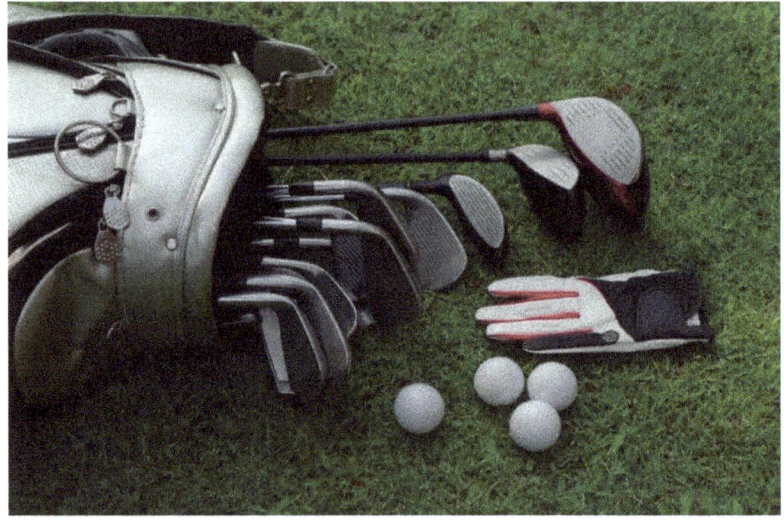

- Drivers: Look for drivers with a larger sweet spot and higher loft (10.5° or more). These features help beginners achieve better accuracy and distance even with less-than-perfect swings. Adjustable drivers can also be beneficial as they allow customization as skills improve.

- o Example: Callaway Rogue ST MAX Driver is highly recommended for its forgiveness and ease of use.

- Irons: Cavity-back irons are best for beginners because they have a larger clubface and perimeter weighting, which increases forgiveness and helps launch the ball higher.

  - o Example: Callaway Rogue ST MAX Irons are beginner-friendly due to their design.

- Wedges: Start with a pitching wedge (PW) and sand wedge (SW). These two wedges cover most short-game scenarios without overwhelming new players.

  - o Example: Cleveland CBX 2 Wedge offers excellent control and forgiveness.

- Putters: Opt for putters with alignment aids to assist in aiming properly on the green. Mallet-style putters are often easier for beginners compared to blade-style putters.

  - o Example: Odyssey White Hot OG Putter is known for its alignment features.

- Complete Sets: For simplicity and cost-effectiveness, consider purchasing a complete beginner set that includes all necessary clubs along with a bag.

  - o Example: Callaway Strata Complete Set is an excellent choice as it provides all essential clubs tailored for new golfers.

## Golf Balls: Focus on Distance and Soft Feel

Choosing the right golf balls can significantly impact performance, especially for beginners who may struggle with both distance and control.

- Distance Balls: These balls are designed to travel farther, making them ideal for players who need extra yardage off the tee.

    o Example: TaylorMade Distance+ Golf Balls offer great value for beginners seeking more distance.

- Soft Feel Balls: For those looking to improve their short game, soft-feel balls provide better control around greens while still offering decent distance.

    o Example: Callaway Supersoft Golf Balls are popular among new golfers due to their forgiving nature.

Beginners should avoid premium tour-level balls as these prioritize spin control over forgiveness, which may not suit novice players' needs.

## Golf Bags: Lightweight and Functional

A good golf bag ensures convenience while carrying or transporting clubs during play. Beginners should choose bags based on how they plan to navigate the course:

- Carry Bags: Lightweight options suitable for walking golfers who prefer minimal weight.

    o Example: Ping Hoofer Lite Carry Bag is easy to carry over long distances.

- Stand Bags: Equipped with built-in stands that keep the bag upright during play; these are versatile options suitable for walking or cart use.

  o Example: Titleist Hybrid 14 Stand Bag combines functionality with ample storage space.

- Cart Bags: Designed specifically for use with golf carts; these bags offer more storage but are heavier than carry or stand bags.

  o Example: Callaway Chev 14 Cart Bag provides stability and plenty of compartments.

# Golf Course Layout

## Golf Basics: Parts of a Golf Course

Golf courses are designed with specific areas that present unique challenges and opportunities for players. Understanding these key parts of a golf course is essential for improving your game, strategizing effectively, and navigating the course successfully. Below is a detailed breakdown of the primary components of a golf course:

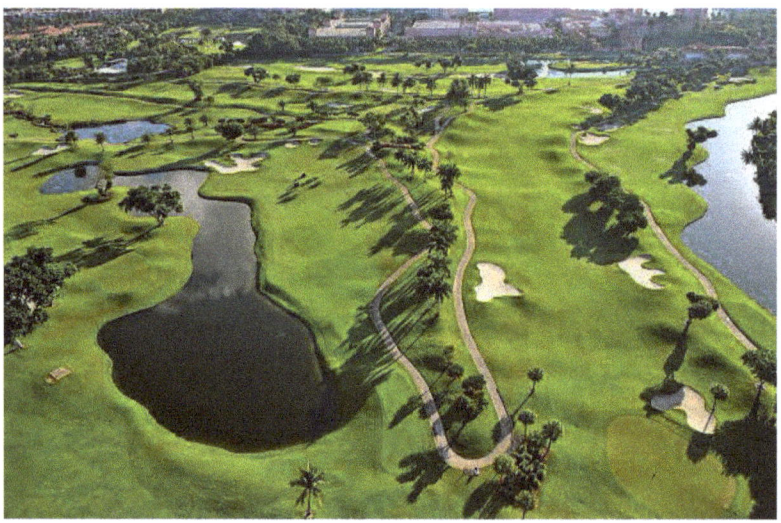

## Tee Boxes

The tee box, also referred to as the teeing ground, marks the starting point for each hole on the course. It is typically a flat area where golfers take their first shot (known as the "tee shot"). Tee boxes are often equipped with markers that indicate where players should place their ball.

- Multiple Tee Options: Most courses have several tee boxes per hole to accommodate different skill levels:

  o Forward tees (closer to the fairway) are designed for beginners or those seeking an easier challenge.

  o Back tees (farthest from the fairway) are intended for advanced players who want to test their skills.

- Rules for Placement: Golfers must place their ball between the two markers and can position it up to two club lengths behind them but never in front of the markers.

## Fairways

The fairway is the stretch of closely mowed grass that connects the tee box to the green. It is considered the ideal landing zone for most shots after teeing off. Fairways provide a smooth surface that makes it easier to hit subsequent shots compared to other areas like roughs or hazards.

- Dimensions: Fairways typically range from 30 to 50 yards in width.

- Grass Types: The type of grass used on fairways varies by region and climate, which can affect gameplay:

  o Bentgrass

  o Ryegrass

  o Bermuda grass

  o Fine fescues

- Strategy: Players aim to land their ball in this area because it allows better control over spin and trajectory when hitting toward the green.

## Greens

The green, also known as the putting green, is where each hole ends. This area contains the cup (hole) and flagstick, which serve as targets for golfers trying to complete each hole.

- Grass Characteristics: The grass on greens is cut extremely short, providing a smooth surface that facilitates rolling putts accurately toward the hole.

- Fringe Area: Surrounding some greens is an area called "the fringe," where grass is slightly longer than on the green itself but shorter than in roughs.

- Reading Greens: Players must assess factors such as slope, grain direction, and moisture levels before putting:

  o Dry greens tend to be faster, causing balls to roll farther.

  o Wet greens slow down ball movement significantly.

## Bunkers/Sand Traps

Bunkers, commonly called sand traps, are depressions filled with sand strategically placed around fairways and greens. They serve as hazards designed to challenge golfers' accuracy and recovery skills.

- Types of Bunkers:

  o Fairway bunkers are located along or near fairways.

  o Greenside bunkers surround putting greens.

- Challenges:
  - Hitting out of bunkers requires specialized techniques such as opening up the clubface and using wedges with high loft angles.
  - Sand consistency can vary depending on weather conditions or course maintenance practices.

## Roughs

The rough refers to areas surrounding fairways and greens where grass is intentionally left longer than in other parts of the course. Roughs add difficulty by making it harder for golfers to hit clean shots due to thicker or taller grass.

- Characteristics:
  - Grass length increases progressively farther away from fairways or greens.
  - Some courses may feature multiple layers of rough with varying heights ("first cut" vs. "deep rough").
- Strategies for Recovery:
  - Use clubs with more loft (e.g., wedges) when hitting out of thick rough.
  - Adjust grip pressure and swing mechanics accordingly.

## Additional Hazards

In addition to bunkers, golf courses often include water hazards such as ponds, lakes, rivers, or creeks. These obstacles further increase difficulty by penalizing errant shots:

**Water Hazards:**

- o Marked with yellow stakes if they cross directly through play areas or red stakes if lateral (alongside play).

- o Players may attempt recovery shots from shallow water but often take penalty strokes instead.

**Out-of-Bounds Areas:**

- o Marked by white stakes; any ball landing here results in penalties requiring replays from previous positions.

By understanding these elements—tee boxes, fairways, greens, bunkers/sand traps, roughs—and how they interact within a golf course layout, players can develop strategies tailored specifically toward minimizing risks while maximizing scoring opportunities.

# Understanding Hole Design

When it comes to understanding golfhole design, the length and layout of each hole play a significant role in shaping the challenge and strategy required for players. Golf courses are designed with a variety of holes to test different aspects of a golfer's skill set, including driving, approach shots, and putting. Below is an in-depth explanation of how holes vary in length and layout.

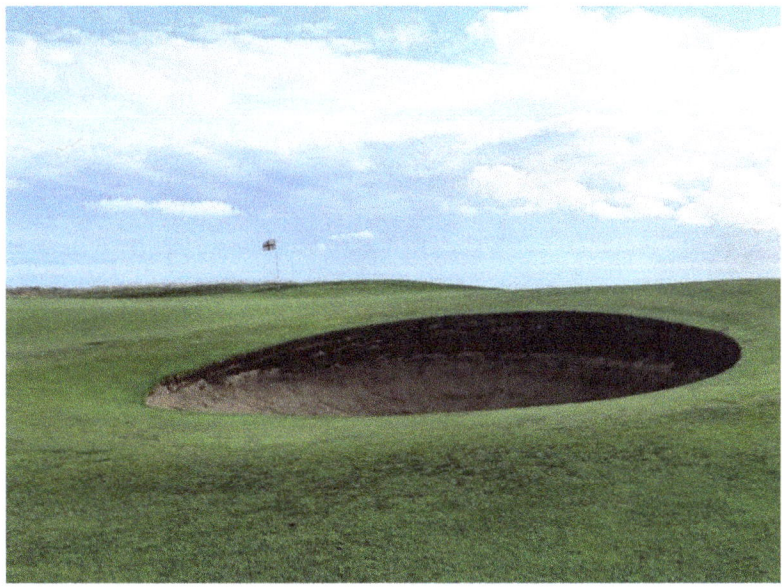

## Hole Length: Par 3s vs. Par 5s

The length of a golf hole is one of the primary factors that determines its classification as a par 3, par 4, or par 5. These classifications are based on the number of strokes an expert golfer (a scratch golfer) is expected to take to complete the hole.

1. Par 3 Holes

- Length: Par 3 holes are typically the shortest on a golf course, ranging from about 90 yards to 240 yards (82 to 220 meters), though most fall between 120 and 200 yards.

- Design Characteristics: Players are expected to reach the green with their tee shot on a par 3. The challenge often lies in accuracy rather than distance, as these holes frequently feature smaller greens or hazards such as bunkers or water near the green.

- Strategy: Precision is key on par 3s since golfers aim directly for the green. Missing the target can result in difficult recovery shots from hazards or rough areas.

2. Par 4 Holes

- While not explicitly part of this question, it's worth noting that par 4s are medium-length holes (typically between 240 and 490 yards) where players generally require two shots to reach the green.

3. Par 5 Holes

- Length: Par 5 holes are longer than par 4s, usually ranging from about 450 yards to over 600 yards (410 to over 550 meters). Some modern courses even feature "monster" par-5 holes exceeding these lengths.

- Design Characteristics: These holes require three strokes for an expert golfer to reach the green under normal conditions— one drive off the tee, one fairway shot, and one approach shot onto the green.

o Strategy: Par-5 holes often provide opportunities for birdies due to their length but also pose challenges with hazards like bunkers or water along their extended fairways. Long hitters may attempt to reach the green in two strokes ("going for it"), but this carries risk if hazards guard the area around the green.

## Hole Layout: Doglegs vs. Straight Holes

In addition to varying lengths, golf hole layouts differ significantly depending on whether they follow a straight path from tee box to green or include bends known as doglegs.

1. Straight Holes

   o Design Characteristics: Straight holes have a direct line from tee box to green without any significant turns or bends in their layout.

   o Strategy: These holes allow golfers to focus primarily on distance and accuracy off the tee without needing to shape their shots around obstacles or corners.

   o Straight layouts can still be challenging if they incorporate elevation changes, narrow fairways bordered by rough or trees, or strategically placed hazards like bunkers and water features.

2. Dogleg Holes

   o Definition: A dogleg refers to a hole that bends either left or right at some point along its fairway—similar in appearance to a dog's hind leg.

     ▪ A "dogleg left" bends leftward after an initial straight section.

- A "dogleg right" bends rightward instead.
  - Design Characteristics: Doglegs add complexity by requiring golfers to adjust their strategy based on how far they can hit their shots and where they want their ball positioned for subsequent shots.
    - For example, players might need to hit shorter clubs off the tee ("laying up") if hitting too far risks overshooting into rough areas beyond the bend.
    - Alternatively, skilled players may attempt "cutting corners" by hitting over trees or other obstacles at sharp angles created by doglegs.
  - Strategy: Success on dogleg holes depends heavily on shot placement and shaping (curving) shots intentionally:
    - A fade (left-to-right ball flight) is useful for dogleg-right holes.
    - A draw (right-to-left ball flight) works well for dogleg-left designs.

## Additional Factors Influencing Hole Design

### Elevation Changes

Holes may feature uphill climbs or downhill slopes that affect both distance and club selection:

- Uphill holes play longer because balls lose momentum traveling upward.
- Downhill holes play shorter as gravity assists ball travel.

## Hazards

Strategically placed hazards such as bunkers (sand traps), water bodies (lakes/streams), and thick rough areas increase difficulty regardless of whether a hole is straight or curved.

## Green Placement

The location of greens relative to surrounding terrain also influences difficulty:

- Elevated greens require precise approaches since balls rolling short won't climb up easily.

- Greens surrounded by bunkers demand accurate landing zones.

By combining variations in length (par values) with diverse layouts like straight paths versus doglegs—and adding elements like elevation changes and hazards—golf architects create unique challenges that test every aspect of a player's game across all types of courses.

# Etiquette

## Etiquette on the Course

Golf is a game deeply rooted in tradition, respect, and courtesy. Beyond the technical rules of play, understanding and adhering to proper golf etiquette is essential for ensuring an enjoyable experience for all players on the course. Below are some key aspects of basic golf etiquette, focusing on repairing divots/ball marks and maintaining pace of play.

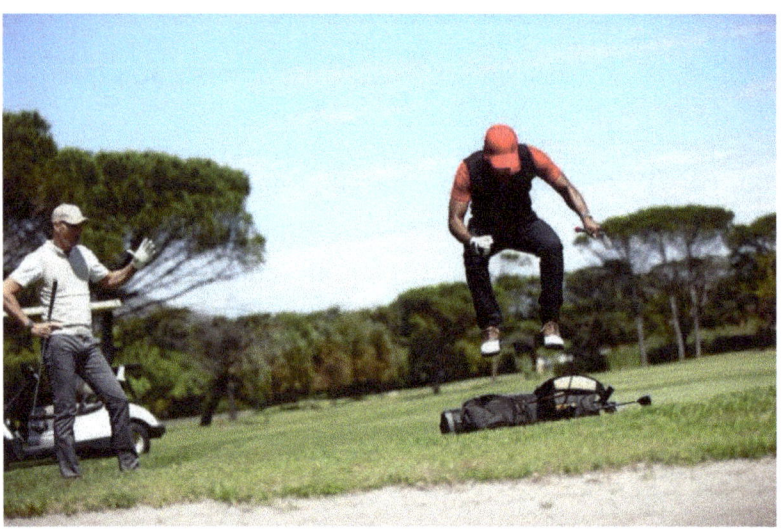

### Repairing Divots and Ball Marks

One of the fundamental principles of golf etiquette is leaving the course in good condition for others. This includes repairing any damage caused during play:

1. Divots: A divot refers to a chunk of turf displaced by a player's club during a swing, typically on fairways or tee boxes. Failing to

repair divots can leave unsightly scars on the course and negatively impact play for others.

- o How to Repair Divots: Replace the dislodged piece of turf back into its original position if possible, pressing it down firmly with your foot or club. Alternatively, many courses provide sand/seed mix that can be used to fill in the damaged area.

- o Why It Matters: Properly repaired divots help maintain healthy grass growth and ensure smooth playing surfaces for subsequent golfers.

2. Ball Marks: These are small indentations left on greens when a ball lands from a height. Unrepaired ball marks can disrupt putting lines and cause long-term damage to the green.

- o How to Repair Ball Marks: Use a ball mark repair tool (or even a tee) to gently lift and push the edges of the indentation back toward the center without tearing the grass roots. Lightly tap down with your putter to smooth out the surface.

- o Why It Matters: Fixing ball marks promptly prevents further deterioration of greens and ensures fair conditions for all players.

# Pace of Play

Maintaining an appropriate pace of play is another critical aspect of golf etiquette. Slow play can lead to frustration among other groups on the course and disrupt overall flow.

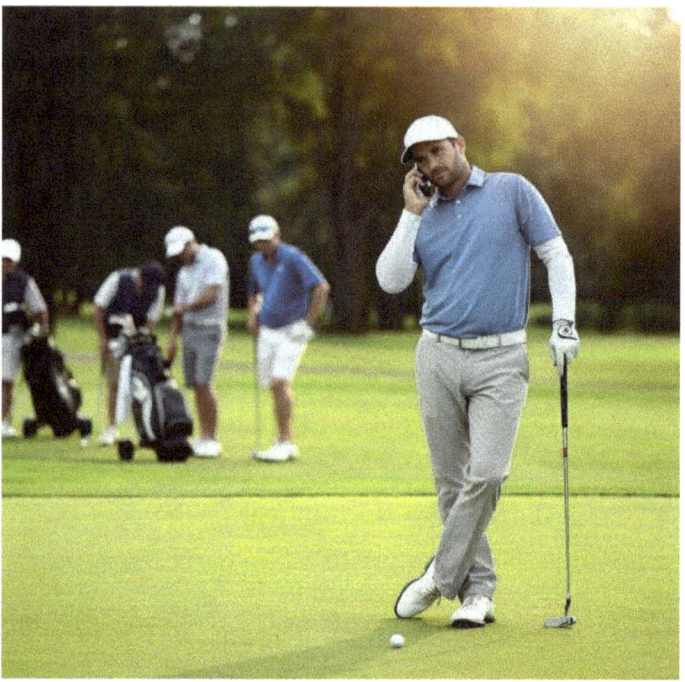

1. Stay Prepared:

   o Be ready to hit your shot when it's your turn by selecting your club in advance and assessing your shot while others are playing.

   o If using a golf cart, park it strategically so you can quickly move between shots without causing delays.

2. Limit Time Spent Searching for Balls:

- o The official rules allow up to three minutes to search for a lost ball; however, if it becomes clear that finding it will take longer, signal the group behind you to "play through" (allow them to pass).

- o Consider carrying extra balls in case one is lost.

3. Play "Ready Golf" When Appropriate:

- o In casual games (as opposed to tournament settings), players should hit their shots as soon as they are ready rather than strictly adhering to who is farthest from the hole.

- o This approach speeds up play while still respecting safety protocols.

4. Let Faster Groups Play Through:

- o If your group is slower than those behind you, allow faster groups to pass by stepping aside at an appropriate point (e.g., after completing a hole or at a tee box). This ensures everyone enjoys their round without unnecessary delays.

5. Keep Up With the Group Ahead:

- o Always aim to maintain pace with the group directly ahead of you rather than focusing solely on those behind you.

- o If there's significant space between your group and those ahead, adjust your speed accordingly or let others pass.

By following these simple guidelines—repairing damage caused during play and keeping pace—you contribute not only to preserving course conditions but also fostering an enjoyable environment for all golfers.

The Journey Begins

# Playing Guidelines

## Play the Ball as It Lies

One of golf's fundamental principles is playing the ball as it lies. This means you cannot move or alter the ball's position unless explicitly allowed by the rules. For example, if your ball lands in a divot or rough terrain, you must play it from that spot unless relief is permitted under specific circumstances.

## Play the Course as You Find It

Similarly, golfers are expected to play the course as they find it without altering its natural state. For instance, breaking branches or smoothing sand in bunkers to gain an advantage is prohibited.

## Out of Bounds and Penalty Areas

If your ball goes out of bounds (marked by white stakes or lines), you must take a one-stroke penalty and replay your shot from its original position. Penalty areas (e.g., water hazards) also incur penalties but offer options such as dropping the ball near where it crossed into the hazard.

## Order of Play

In stroke play, the player with the lowest score on the previous hole tees off first ("honors"). During play on each hole, the golfer farthest from the hole plays next.

## Relief Options

Relief can be taken in certain situations like abnormal course conditions (e.g., ground under repair) or obstructions (e.g., cart paths).

Depending on circumstances, relief may involve dropping your ball within a designated area without penalty.

## Scoring Formats

Golf has two primary formats: match play (competing hole-by-hole) and stroke play (total strokes over 18 holes). Understanding which format you're playing ensures proper scoring and competition flow.

## Penalties

Penalties are incurred for rule violations such as hitting out of bounds or grounding your club in a bunker before striking the ball. These typically add one or two strokes to your score depending on severity.

# Basic Rules About Penalties

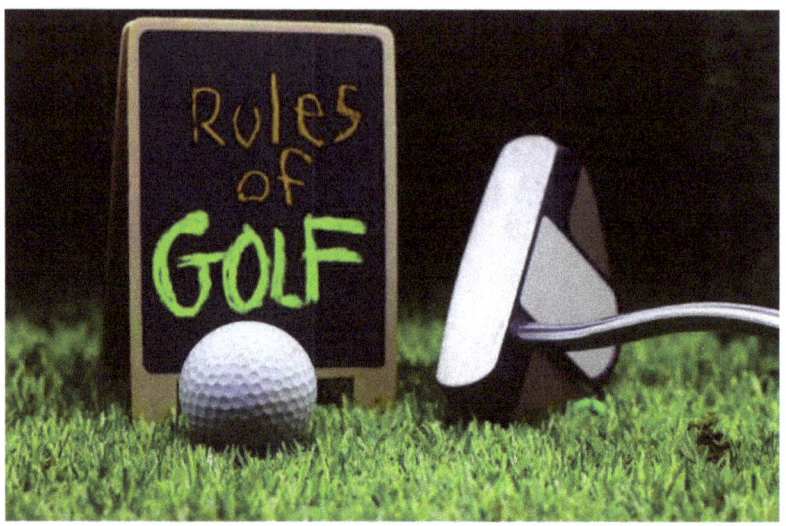

Golf is a game governed by a comprehensive set of rules, and penalties are an integral part of ensuring fair play. Below is a detailed explanation of the basic rules regarding penalties for common situations like out-of-bounds shots and water hazards.

## Out-of-Bounds Shots

An "out-of-bounds" (OB) area is defined as any part of the course that lies outside the boundaries marked by white stakes or lines. When a ball goes out of bounds, the following rules apply:

1. **Penalty Stroke**: The player incurs a one-stroke penalty.

2. **Stroke-and-Distance Rule**: The player must replay the shot from the original spot where they last played (this is referred to as "stroke-and-distance"). For example:

o   If your tee shot goes out of bounds, you must hit another ball from the tee box, which will now be your third stroke.

3. **Provisional Ball Option**: To save time, players can declare and play a provisional ball if they suspect their original ball may be out of bounds. If the original ball is found in bounds, it must be played, and the provisional ball is disregarded.

It's important to note that local rules may sometimes allow alternative options for OB relief (e.g., dropping near where the ball went out with additional penalties), but these are not standard under USGA or R&A Rules.

## Water Hazards

Water hazards are areas on the course marked specifically as either yellow or red hazards. Each type has distinct relief options:

### Yellow Water Hazards

These are typically regular water hazards that require playing over or around them. When a ball enters a yellow hazard, players have three options:

1. **Play It As It Lies**: If possible, you can attempt to hit your ball from within the hazard without penalty.

2. **Stroke-and-Distance Relief**: Replay your shot from where you last played it with a one-stroke penalty.

3. **Back-on-the-Line Relief**: Drop a new ball on an imaginary straight line extending back from the hole through the point where your ball last crossed into the hazard. You can go as far back along this line as you wish but incur a one-stroke penalty.

**Red Water Hazards [Lateral Hazards]**

Red hazards are lateral water hazards often running alongside fairways or greens. In addition to all yellow hazard relief options above, red hazards provide two additional relief choices:

1. **Two Club-Lengths Relief**: Drop within two club-lengths of where your ball last crossed into the hazard, no closer to the hole, with a one-stroke penalty.

2. **Opposite Side Relief**: Drop within two club-lengths on the opposite side of the hazard at an equidistant point from where your ball entered, no closer to the hole, with a one-stroke penalty.

## General Notes on Penalty Strokes

- Penalty strokes do not count as physical swings but are added to your score for that hole.

- Always confirm whether local rules or tournament-specific guidelines modify standard procedures for OB or water hazards.

- Players should mark their balls clearly and pay attention to markings on stakes/lines (white for OB, yellow/red for water hazards) to avoid confusion during play.

By understanding these basic rules about penalties in golf, players can navigate challenging situations more effectively while adhering to proper etiquette and regulations.

# Fundamentals: Set Up Through Finish

The golf swing is a complex motion that requires coordination, balance, and proper mechanics to achieve consistent results. The fundamentals of swing mechanics include several key components: grip, stance, posture, alignment, backswing, downswing, and follow-through. Each element plays a critical role in ensuring a smooth and effective swing.

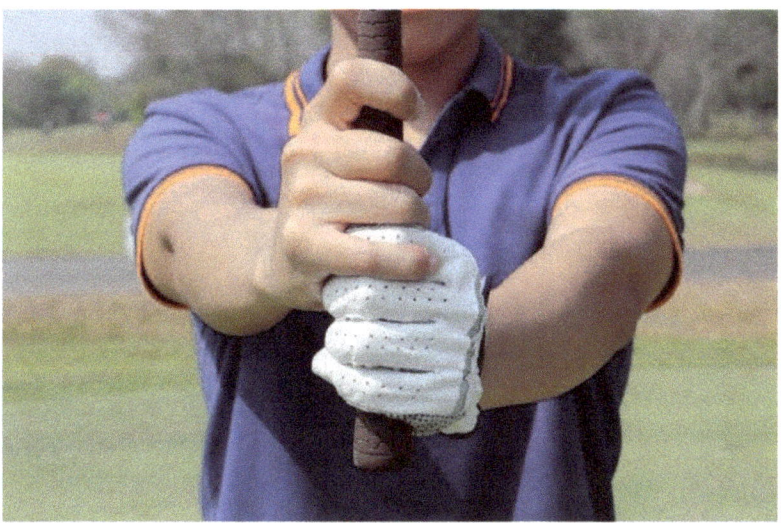

## Proper Grip Techniques

### Overlapping Grip or Interlocking Grip

The grip is one of the most fundamental aspects of a golfer's setup because it directly influences the control and power of the swing. A proper grip ensures that the hands work together as a single unit during the swing while maintaining control over the clubface. Here are two widely used grip techniques:

Overlapping Grip (Vardon Grip): The overlapping grip is the most commonly used grip among professional golfers and is often taught to beginners with larger hands. It was popularized by Harry Vardon in the early 20th century and remains a standard technique in golf instruction today.

**How to Perform the Overlapping Grip:**

- Start by holding the club with your left hand (for right-handed golfers). Place the club handle diagonally across your fingers rather than in your palm.

- Wrap your left hand around the club so that your thumb points down along the shaft.

- Position your right hand below your left hand on the club.

- Lift your right pinky finger and rest it on top of or between the index and middle fingers of your left hand.

- Ensure there is no gap between your hands; they should feel unified.

**Advantages:**

- Provides better control over wrist movement during the swing.

- Helps unify both hands for improved consistency.

- Ideal for players with larger hands or longer fingers.

**Disadvantages:**

- May feel unnatural for beginners at first.

- Requires practice to develop comfort and effectiveness.

Interlocking Grip: The interlocking grip is another popular technique, especially among players with smaller hands or shorter fingers. This method involves physically linking one finger from each hand to create a secure connection between them.

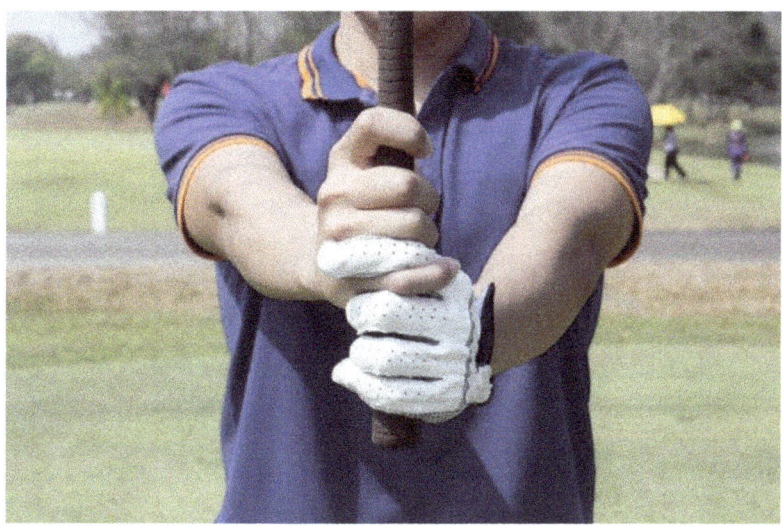

**How to Perform the Interlocking Grip:**

1. Begin by gripping the club with your left hand as described above for right-handed golfers.

2. Place your right hand below your left on the club handle.

3. Interlock your right pinky finger with your left index finger so they are securely linked together.

4. Wrap both hands around the club so they feel connected and stable.

**Advantages:**

- Provides an even stronger connection between both hands compared to other grips.

- Reduces independent movement of each hand during the swing, promoting consistency.

- Favored by some of golf's greatest players, including Tiger Woods and Jack Nicklaus.

**Disadvantages:**

- Can feel restrictive for players who prefer more freedom in their wrist action.

- May not be comfortable for those with larger hands or limited flexibility.

Both grips have their merits but choosing between them depends on individual preferences such as hand size, comfort level, and personal playing style.

# Stance and Posture

## How to stand correctly with balance and alignment

### Fundamentals of Swing Mechanics

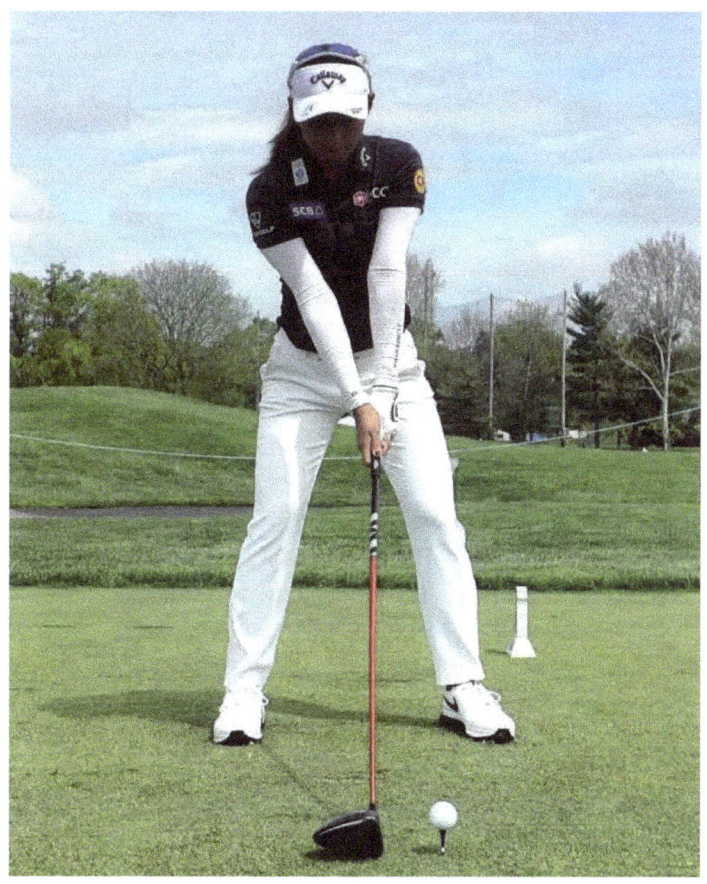

To achieve a correct stance and posture in golf, it is essential to focus on balance, alignment, and proper body positioning. These elements form the foundation for a consistent and powerful swing. Below is a

The Journey Begins

detailed explanation of how to stand correctly with balance and alignment:

**Foot Positioning and Width of Stance**

o Begin by placing your feet shoulder-width apart. This width provides a stable base while allowing for proper weight transfer during the swing.

o Your feet should be parallel to the target line (the imaginary line running from your ball to your intended target). This ensures that your body is aligned properly toward the target.

**Ball Position**

o The position of the ball relative to your stance depends on the club you are using:

  ▪ For longer clubs like drivers, place the ball slightly forward in your stance, near your lead foot (left foot for right-handed golfers).

  ▪ For mid-irons, position the ball just forward of center.

  ▪ For shorter irons or wedges, place the ball closer to the center of your stance.

**Weight Distribution**

o Distribute your weight evenly between both feet at address (the starting position before you begin your swing). Avoid leaning too far forward onto your toes or backward onto your heels.

o Your weight should feel balanced over your ankles, which helps maintain stability throughout the swing.

**Knee Flexion and Hip Hinge**

o Slightly flex your knees—not too much or too little—to create an athletic posture. This slight bend allows for better mobility during the swing.

o Bend from your hips rather than rounding your back or slouching forward. To do this correctly:

  ▪ Keep a straight spine as you hinge forward from the hips.

  ▪ Let gravity naturally lower your upper body toward the ball while maintaining good posture.

**Back and Shoulder Alignment**

o Your back should remain straight but not rigid—maintain a natural curve in your lower spine.

o Align your shoulders parallel to the target line. If they tilt excessively up or down, it can cause poor angles that disrupt balance and lead to inconsistent shots.

**Head Position**

o Keep your head slightly behind the ball at address (especially for longer clubs like drivers). This positioning, known as the Reverse K, helps promote an upward strike on drives while maintaining balance.

o Avoid tucking or lifting your chin excessively; keep it neutral so that you can rotate freely during the swing.

**Arm Position and Relaxation**

o Let your arms hang naturally from their sockets without tension.

o Keep both elbows straight and close together.

**Alignment Checkpoints to ensure proper alignment:**

o Your hips, knees, shoulders, and feet should all be aligned parallel to each other and perpendicular to the target line.

o Use visual aids like alignment sticks during practice sessions to confirm that everything is lined up correctly.

**Final posture check before swinging before initiating any movement:**

o Ensure that you feel balanced over both feet with no excessive leaning in any direction.

o Confirm that there's no excessive shaft lean—your hands should be slightly ahead of or level with the ball at address but not overly tilted forward.

By following these steps consistently, you will establish a solid setup position that promotes balance, alignment, and power throughout every phase of the golf swing.

# The Proper Golf Swing

The golf swing is a complex motion that can be broken down into three main components: the **backswing**, **downswing**, and **follow-through**. Each part plays a critical role in ensuring a consistent, powerful, and accurate shot. Below is a detailed explanation of each phase of the swing process.

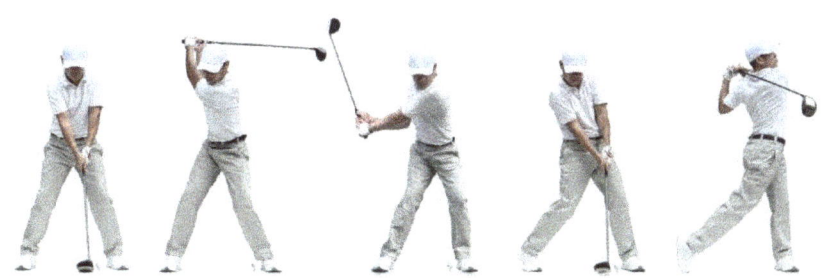

## The Swing Process

### Backswing

The backswing is the initial movement where you prepare to generate power for your shot. It involves moving the club away from the ball while maintaining proper alignment and balance. Here are the key steps:

1. **Takeaway**: Start by moving the club back in one piece, keeping your arms, hands, and chest connected as a unit. The club should remain low to the ground during this phase.

2. **Rotation**: Rotate your shoulders around your spine while keeping your lower body stable. Your weight should gradually shift to your back foot (right foot for right-handed players).

3. **Arm Position**: As you lift the club, ensure that your lead arm (left arm for right-handed golfers) stays straight but not rigid. Your trail arm (right arm) will naturally bend at the elbow.

4. **Club Position at the Top**: At the top of your backswing, your hands should be above or slightly behind your head, with the club pointing roughly parallel to the target line.

**Key Thought: Maintain a smooth tempo throughout the backswing and avoid rushing this step.**

**Downswing**

The downswing is where you transition from storing energy in your backswing to releasing it into the ball for maximum impact. This phase requires coordination between your upper and lower body.

1. **Initiation**: The downswing begins with a slight shift of weight from your back foot to your front foot (left foot for right-handed players). This movement starts with your hips rather than your arms or shoulders.

2. **Hip Rotation**: As you rotate through impact, allow your hips to lead while keeping your upper body slightly behind them. This creates lag—a key factor in generating power.

3. **Club Path**: Ensure that the club follows an inside-to-outside path relative to the target line as it approaches impact.

4. **Impact Position**: At impact, most of your weight should be on your front foot, with both arms extended toward the target and wrists unhinging naturally.

**Key Thought: Focus on maintaining control during this phase— power comes from proper sequencing rather than brute force.**

## Follow-Through

The follow-through completes the swing and ensures that all energy has been transferred into the ball effectively while maintaining balance.

1. **Extension**: After striking the ball, continue extending both arms toward the target as long as possible before they begin folding naturally.

2. **Body Rotation**: Your torso should fully rotate so that your chest faces toward the target at completion.

3. **Finish Position**: End with most of your weight on your front foot, standing tall with good posture and balance.

**Key Thought: A balanced finish position indicates that you maintained control throughout all phases of the swing.**

# Short Game Skills

## Putting Basics

### How to read greens

Reading greens is an essential skill for putting success in golf. It involves analyzing various factors that influence how a ball will roll on its way to the hole. Below are detailed steps and techniques for mastering this skill:

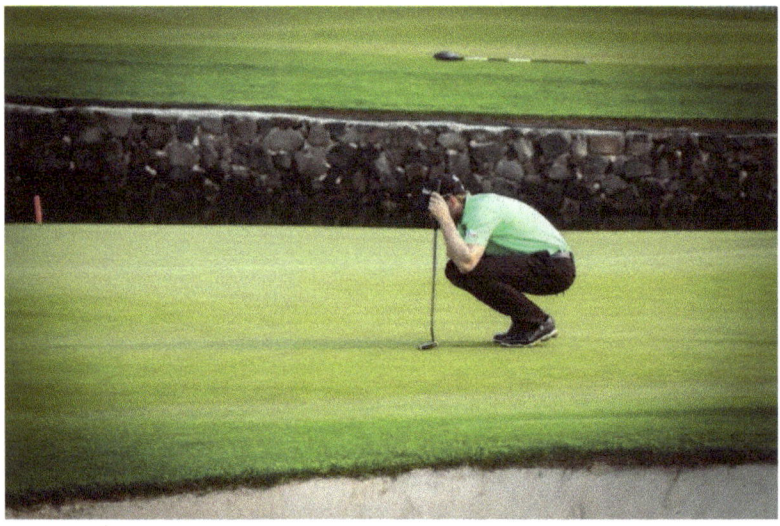

### Assessing Overall Terrain

- Walk around the green to observe its general layout.

- Look for slopes, ridges, valleys, or any noticeable contours that could affect ball movement.

- Imagine pouring water onto the green—where it would flow indicates low points where putts may break toward.

**Understanding Grass Grain**

- Grass grain refers to the direction in which grass grows on a green:

    o Lighter patches indicate grass growing away from you (faster putts).

    o Darker patches indicate grass growing toward you (slower putts).

- Grain direction can subtly alter both speed and break.

**Analyzing Surroundings**

- Environmental factors such as sunlight and shadows can distort perception:

    o Shadows may exaggerate slopes or breaks.

    o Consider wind direction if it's strong enough to influence putts.

**Using Green Reading Technique**

Several methods can help golfers better understand breaks and slopes:

- **Plumb-Bob Method:** Hold your putter vertically in front of you while standing behind the ball; observe how it aligns with slopes relative to the hole.

- **Aimpoint Putting Method:** Use fingers held up against slopes behind the ball to gauge break severity (requires training but offers precise results).

**Identifying High Points**

Every putt has a "high point"—the spot where gravity begins pulling it toward its final path:

- Crouch down behind both ball and hole at eye level with each slope section.

- Aim slightly above this high point so gravity assists rather than hinders progress toward sinking putts.

**Adjusting for Speed**

Speed determines how much break affects a putt

- Faster putts break less because they travel straighter over shorter distances before slowing down.

- Slower putts break more due to prolonged exposure time across sloped surfaces.

**Visualizing Ball Path**

Before executing any stroke

- Mentally trace an ideal path from start-to-finish based upon terrain analysis above combined w/ chosen pace preferences beforehand.

# **Putting Stroke**

Putting requires precision rather than power, making its mechanics distinct from full-swing techniques:

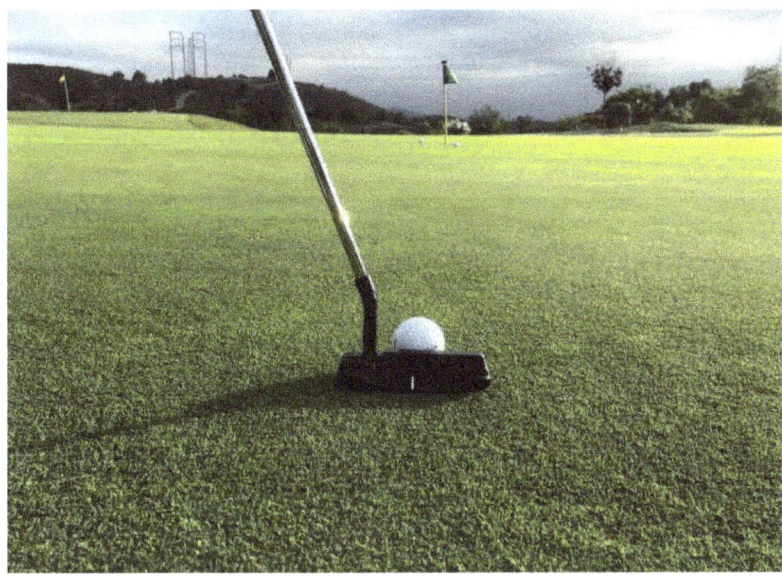

Shoulder Dominance: The putting stroke relies primarily on rocking shoulders back-and-forth like pendulum motion instead of involving wrists/arms independently moving around themselves unnecessarily complicating process overall execution consistency suffers greatly otherwise.

Lower Body Stability: Keep legs still throughout entire stroke sequence ensuring no unnecessary movements disrupt rhythm/cadence established beforehand.

## Proper Putting Stroke Technique

A proper putting stroke is essential for consistent performance on the greens in golf. It involves a combination of physical setup, stroke mechanics, and mental focus. Below are the key components of a proper putting stroke technique broken down step by step:

### 1. Setup and Posture

The foundation of a good putting stroke begins with your setup and posture. Proper alignment and comfort are crucial to ensure consistency.

- Weight Distribution: Your weight should be evenly balanced on both feet. This creates skeletal alignment, which stabilizes your body and reduces tension during the stroke.

- Ball Position: Place the ball slightly forward in your stance, just ahead of the centerline. This ensures that you strike the ball on the upward part of your putting arc, promoting a smooth roll.

- Posture Check: Bend slightly at the hips so that your arms hang naturally without excessive bending or stiffness. A good rule of thumb is to tilt forward until your fingertips touch the top of your kneecaps before gripping the putter.

- Grip Consistency: While there are various grip styles (e.g., traditional, claw, cross-handed), maintaining a consistent grip is more important than the specific style you choose. A stable grip helps control wrist movement and keeps your putter face square.

### 2. Stroke Mechanics

The actual motion of the putting stroke should be smooth, controlled and repeatable.

- Tempo: The tempo of your putting stroke should follow a 1:1 ratio—your forward swing should be exactly the same as your backswing. This rhythm ensures consistency in distance control.

- Putter Path: While many golfers aim for a "straight back, straight through" motion, it's natural for the putter to follow a slight arc due to body mechanics. Trying too hard to force a perfectly straight path can lead to inconsistencies.

- Wrist Movement Control: Limit excessive wrist motion during the stroke. While some minor wrist movement occurs naturally due to gravity and momentum, keeping it minimal ensures better control over direction and distance.

## 3. Key Focus Areas During Stroke

To execute an effective putting stroke consistently, focus on these critical elements:

- Let Gravity Work: Avoid forcing or jamming the putter through impact. Instead, let gravity guide the putter head naturally during both backswing and downswing.

- Head Position: Keep your head down throughout the entire stroke until well after impact. Lifting your head too early disrupts posture and can cause miss-hits.

- Smooth Transition: Ensure there's no jerky movement between setup and backswing initiation; this helps maintain balance throughout.

## 4. Practice Drills for Improvement

Practicing specific drills can help refine your putting technique:

- Metronome Drill for Tempo: Use a metronome set at 72–80 beats per minute to practice maintaining a consistent 1:1 tempo ratio in both short and long putts.

- Gate Drill for Putter Path Control: Set up two tees slightly wider than your putter head along its intended path; practice stroking without hitting either tee.

## 5. Mental Approach

Putting is as much about mental focus as physical execution:

- Visualize success before each putt by imagining how it will roll into the hole.

- Stay confident even after missed attempts—confidence breeds consistency over time.

By mastering these aspects—setup, mechanics, focus areas, drills, and mental preparation—you'll develop a reliable putting stroke that improves accuracy and lowers scores.

# Chipping

Chipping is a low trajectory shot played close to the green, where the ball spends minimal time in the air and rolls out toward the hole. It is often used when there are no significant obstacles between the ball and the target.

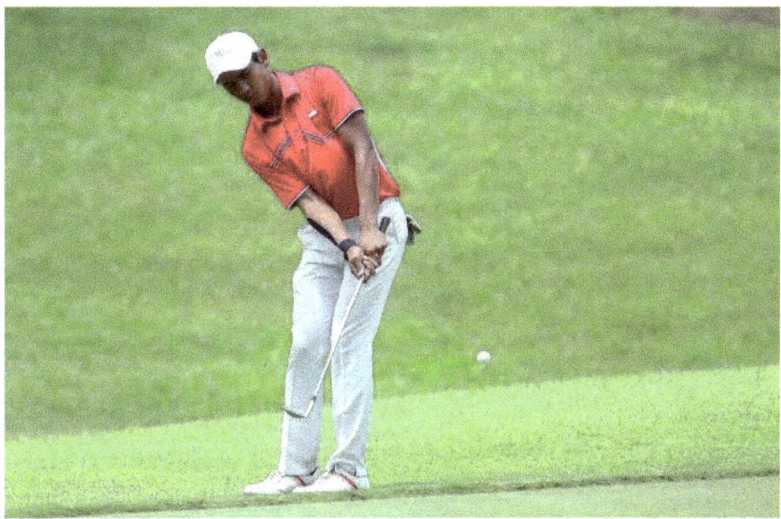

## Key Characteristics:

1. Trajectory and Roll: The ball travels low to the ground with limited airtime and relies heavily on rolling after landing.

2. Distance: Typically used for short distances, usually just off the green or within a few yards of it.

3. Clubs Used: A variety of clubs can be used for chipping, ranging from wedges (pitching wedge) to lower-lofted irons like a 7-iron or even hybrids, depending on how much roll is desired.

## Technique:

### Stance and Setup:

- o   Narrow stance with feet about 4 to 6 inches foot apart.

- o   Weight distributed more on the lead foot (about 70%).

- o   Ball positioned off lead or trail foot depending on loft needed: lead is higher and trail is lower.

- o   Hands ahead of the ball with a slight forward shaft lean.

### Swing Motion:

- o   Similar to a putting stroke, using mostly shoulders with minimal wrist movement.

- o   Keep hands firm and avoid excessive wrist hinge.

- o   Maintain smooth acceleration through impact without deceleration.

### Landing Point Focus:

Visualize where you want the ball to land (typically about 20% of the way to the hole) so it rolls out properly toward your target.

# Pitching

Definition: Pitching is a higher-trajectory shot designed to carry over obstacles such as bunkers or rough before landing softly on the green with minimal roll-out. It is used when more airtime is required than what a chip shot provides.

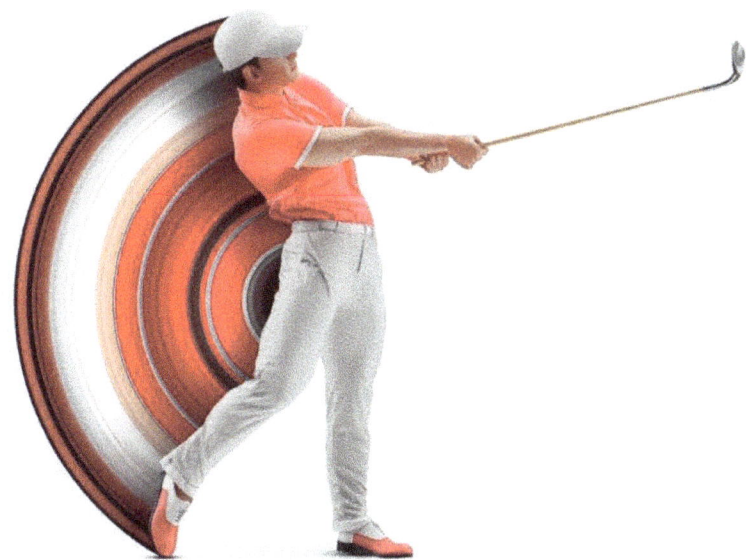

## Key Characteristics:

1. Trajectory and Roll: The ball travels higher in the air compared to a chip shot and has less roll after landing due to its steeper descent angle.

2. Distance: Typically used for slightly longer distances than chips, ranging up to around 30 yards from the green.

3. Clubs Used: Higher-lofted clubs like sand wedges (54°–56°), lob wedges (58°–60°), or gap wedges are ideal for pitching.

## Technique:

### Stance and Setup:

- ○ Slightly wider stance compared to chipping but still narrower than for full swings.

- ○ Weight remains slightly favoring your lead foot but more balanced than during chipping.

- ○ Ball positioned near the center of your stance for consistent contact.

### Swing Motion:

- ○ A pitch shot involves more wrist hinge than a chip shot, resembling a mini version of your full swing.

- ○ Use soft grip pressure and allow your wrists to hinge naturally during backswing while maintaining control over clubface alignment.

- ○ Turn your body away from and then toward the target during backswing and follow-through, ensuring weight transfer occurs smoothly within this smaller range of motion.

### Follow Through:

Finish high with good acceleration through impact; avoid deceleration as it can lead to poor contact or inconsistent results.

Pitch when you need to carry over an obstacle such as rough, bunkers, or water hazards near the green.

When you require more height on your shot for softer landings that minimize roll-out.

Key Differences Between Chipping & Pitching

| Aspect | Chipping | Pitching |
|---|---|---|
| Trajectory | Low | High |
| Roll After Landing | Significant | Minimal |
| Distance | Very short (close proximity) | Slightly longer (up to ~30 yards) |
| Clubs Used | Lower lofted clubs (7–9 iron, pitching wedge) | Higher lofted clubs (sand/lob/gap wedge) |
| Technique | Putting-like stroke with firm wrists | Mini swing with wrist hinge |

# Chipping vs. Pitching

Understanding when to chip versus when to pitch is crucial for improving your short game and lowering your scores. These two shots serve different purposes and are used in distinct scenarios based on the distance, obstacles, and desired ball trajectory. Below is a detailed explanation of when to use each shot.

## When to Chip

Chipping is typically used when you are close to the green and there are no significant obstacles between you and the hole. The goal of a chip shot is to keep the ball low, allowing it to roll out toward the target like a putt after minimal airtime. Here are the key situations where chipping is appropriate:

1. Proximity to the Green: Use a chip shot when you are within a few yards of the green, especially if you only need minimal carry before letting the ball roll.

2. No Obstacles: If there are no hazards such as bunkers, rough, or water between you and the hole, chipping is ideal since it minimizes risk.

3. Flat Terrain: Chipping works best on flat or slightly sloped areas where you can predict how the ball will roll after landing.

4. Control Over Distance: A chip shot provides more control over distance because it uses a putting-like stroke with minimal wrist action.

5. Club Selection: You can use various clubs for chipping depending on how much roll you want—ranging from wedges (for less roll) to lower-lofted clubs like 7-irons or hybrids (for more roll).

## When to Pitch

Pitching is used when you need more airtime for your shot due to obstacles or longer distances from the green. The pitch shot has a higher trajectory than a chip shot and lands softly with less roll upon impact. Here's when pitching should be employed:

1. Obstacles Between You and the Hole: If there's a bunker, rough, water hazard, or other obstacle that requires carrying the ball over it, pitching is necessary.

2. Longer Distances from the Green: Pitch shots are effective for distances up to around 30 yards where rolling the ball isn't feasible.

3. Uneven Lies or Slopes: When dealing with uneven terrain or slopes near the green, pitching helps ensure better control over where your ball lands.

4. Heavy Rough: In thick grass or deep rough near the green, using a higher-lofted club for pitching allows you to lift the ball out cleanly without excessive resistance from vegetation.

5. High Trajectory Needed: When you need height in your shot— such as clearing an obstacle—or want minimal rollout after landing (e.g., stopping quickly on firm greens), pitching is preferred.

## Key Differences Between Chipping and Pitching

- Trajectory: Chips have low trajectories with more roll; pitches have high trajectories with less roll.

- Distance Covered in Air vs Ground Roll:

  - Chips spend most of their time rolling along the ground after landing.

  - Pitches travel farther through the air before landing softly with limited rollout.

- Club Selection:

  - Chips can be played with various clubs (7-iron through wedges).

  - Pitches require higher-lofted clubs like sand wedges (54–56 degrees) or lob wedges (58–60 degrees).

- Swing Mechanics:

  - Chipping involves minimal wrist hinge and resembles a putting stroke.

  - Pitching uses wrist hinge and body rotation similar to a smaller version of a full swing.

In general:

- Use chipping whenever possible because it's simpler, lower-risk, and easier to control due to its compact motion resembling putting.

- Reserve pitching for situations that require height, carry over obstacles, or soft landings on challenging terrain.

By understanding these distinctions and practicing both techniques regularly, golfers can make smarter decisions around greens and improve their overall scoring potential.

The Journey Begins

# Short Game Drills for Accuracy

Improving accuracy in your short game is essential to lowering your scores and becoming a more consistent golfer. Below are detailed drills designed to enhance precision in different aspects of the short game, from chipping to pitching and bunker play. These drills focus on developing touch, control, and consistency.

## 1. Ladder Drill for Distance Control

This drill helps you improve accuracy by focusing on controlling the distance of your shots, which is critical for precise placement around the green.

**How to Perform:**

1. Place five alignment sticks or tees at intervals of 5 yards starting from 10 yards away (e.g., at 10, 15, 20, 25, and 30 yards).

2. Using a wedge (sand wedge or lob wedge), hit shots aiming to land the ball as close as possible to each marker.

3. Start with the closest target and work your way back to the farthest one.

**Focus Points:**

1. Pay attention to the length of your backswing for each distance.

2. Use smooth tempo and consistent contact.

3. Track how many attempts it takes you to hit each target accurately.

- Why It Works: This drill trains you to control trajectory and spin while improving your ability to judge distances.

## 2. Circle Drill for Chipping Accuracy

The circle drill is excellent for improving accuracy when chipping onto the green and getting up-and-down more often.

**How to Perform:**

1. Select a hole on the practice green and place four tees in a circle around it, each about three feet away from the hole.

2. From various spots around the green (e.g., rough, fringe), chip balls toward the hole aiming to stop them within this three-foot circle.

3. Repeat this process from different distances (5 yards, 10 yards, etc.).

**Focus Points:**

1. Focus on landing spots rather than just aiming at the hole.

2. Use proper technique with soft hands and minimal wrist hinge.

3. Experiment with different clubs (e.g., pitching wedge vs. sand wedge) based on shot requirements.

- Why It Works: This drill improves both landing spot precision and rollout control, helping you consistently leave yourself makeable putts.

## 3. Gate Drill for Clubface Control

This drill focuses on ensuring that your clubface remains square through impact for accurate direction control during chips or pitches.

**How to Perform:**

1. Place two alignment sticks or clubs parallel on either side of your intended target line about six inches apart (forming a "gate").

2. Set up a ball between these sticks and practice hitting chip shots through the gate without touching either stick.

**Focus Points:**

1. Keep your swing path straight through impact.

2. Maintain a steady rhythm with no excessive wrist movement.

- Why It Works: The gate drill ensures that you are striking chips with proper alignment and clubface control, leading to straighter shots.

## 4. High-Low Target Drill for Versatility

This drill enhances accuracy by teaching you how to hit both high-lofted shots that stop quickly and low bump-and-run shots that roll out toward their target.

**How to Perform:**

1. Choose two targets on the practice green—one closer requiring a high shot with soft landing, and one farther requiring a lower trajectory shot that rolls out.

2. Alternate between hitting high lofted shots using a lob wedge or sand wedge for closer targets and bump-and-run shots using an iron (e.g., an 8-iron) for farther targets.

**Focus Points:**

1. For high shots: Open your stance slightly with an open clubface; use a steeper angle of attack.

2. For low shots: Use minimal wrist action with weight slightly forward; focus on clean contact.

Why It Works: This drill builds versatility in shot selection while improving directional accuracy under varying conditions.

## 5. Clock Face Putting Drill

Although primarily focused on putting accuracy, this drill also benefits short-game scenarios where precise placement near holes is required after chips or pitches.

**How to Perform:**

1. Place tees around a hole in positions resembling numbers on a clock face (at equal distances like three feet).

2. Chip balls toward these positions aiming either directly into holes or stopping them close enough within tap-in range depending upon difficulty level chosen!

Why Effective? Builds confidence handling pressure situations needing pinpoint placements.

## Adjustments for Different Lies

Not all chip shots are played from perfect lies; therefore, adjustments must be made depending on where the ball is positioned.

**Ball in Thick Rough or Depression:**

o Move the ball back in your stance (closer to your trail foot).

- Lean more weight onto your lead side and keep it there throughout the swing.

- Use a steeper angle of attack by striking down on the ball with minimal wrist hinge.

- Focus on contacting the ball first while avoiding excessive grass interference.

**Ball Nestled Down in Rough:**

- Use a higher-lofted wedge (e.g., sand wedge or lob wedge) to help lift the ball out of its position.

- Keep shoulders level and avoid leaning back during impact—this ensures you don't "scoop" at the ball.

- Maintain consistent rhythm

**High Lofted Shots for Soft Landings**

When you need to hit a high shot that lands softly (e.g., over an obstacle or onto a fast green), additional loft and technique adjustments are required.

**Setup**:

- Position the ball slightly forward in your stance (closer to your lead foot).

- Open both your stance and clubface slightly—this increases loft while promoting spin.

**Swing Mechanics**:

- Incorporate more wrist hinge during the backswing to create additional height.

○ Allow gravity to drop the clubhead under the ball during impact without forcing it upward.

**Key Tip**:

○ Avoid decelerating through impact; maintain smooth acceleration for consistent results.

**Controlling Distance**

Distance control is one of the most challenging aspects of short shots around the green but can be improved with practice:

- Use varying lengths of backswing depending on how far you want to hit each shot. A shorter backswing produces less power, while a longer one generates more distance.

- Practice rhythm by imagining smooth motions like "putting with loft." This helps create consistency without overthinking mechanics.

# Common Mistakes and How To Avoid Them

Many golfers struggle with short shots due to improper technique or misconceptions about how these shots should be executed:

- **Mistake: Trying to Lift The Ball Into The Air**

Solution: Trust that lofted clubs will naturally elevate the ball when struck correctly. Focus instead on striking down slightly through impact.

- **Mistake: Overusing Wrists During Swing**

Solution: Minimize wrist action by keeping hands quiet during shorter chips; let body rotation guide movement instead.

The Journey Begins

- **Mistake: Decelerating Through Impact**

Solution: Always accelerate smoothly through impact—even on delicate shots—to avoid chunking or thinning.

## Practicing Short Game Techniques

To improve consistency around greens, structured practice is essential:

1. Start by practicing basic chip-and-run shots from flat lies before progressing to more challenging scenarios like uphill/downhill lies or thick rough.

2. Experiment with different clubs (e.g., pitching wedge vs lob wedge) for various trajectories and rollouts.

3. Use drills such as landing balls within specific target zones marked on greens or mats—this builds precision over time.

# Driving & Longer Shots

## How to Hit Off the Tee Using a Driver

Hitting off the tee with a driver is one of the most critical skills in golf, as it sets up your position for the rest of the hole. A consistent and accurate drive can help you find more fairways, improve your scoring potential, and build confidence. Below is a detailed step-by-step guide on how to hit off the tee using a driver effectively:

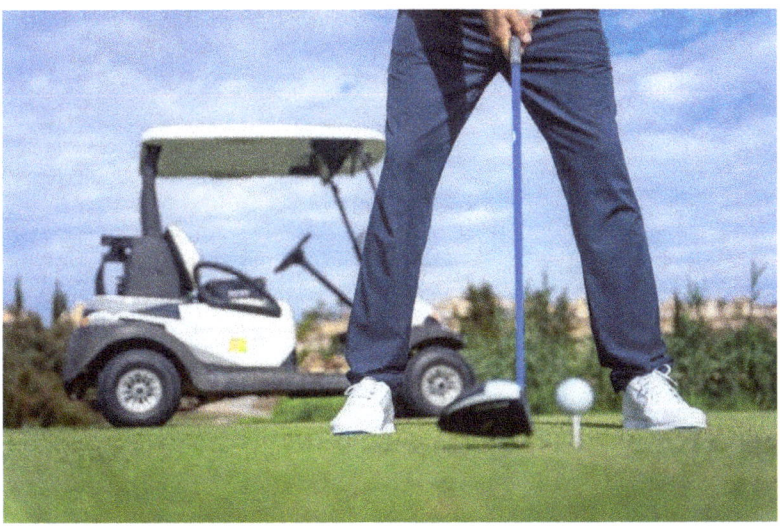

### 1. Set Up Properly

The foundation of a good drive starts with your setup. Here's how to do it correctly:

- Ball Position: Place the ball just inside your front heel (left heel for right-handed golfers). This forward ball position allows you to strike the ball on an upward angle, which is crucial for maximizing distance and achieving optimal launch conditions.

- Tee Height: Adjust the height of your tee so that half of the golf ball sits above the top edge of your driver clubface when addressing it. This ensures you make contact slightly above the center of the clubface, promoting higher launch and lower spin.

- Stance Width: Your feet should be shoulder-width apart or slightly wider. A stable base helps generate power while maintaining balance throughout your swing.

- Posture: Stand tall but tilt your spine slightly away from the target (toward your trail side). This tilt promotes an upward angle of attack during impact.

- Grip Pressure: Hold the club with moderate grip pressure—firm enough to control it but not so tight that it restricts wrist movement or creates tension in your arms.

## 2. Focus on Your Backswing

A proper backswing sets up a powerful downswing and clean contact:

- Shoulder Turn: Rotate your shoulders fully while keeping your lower body stable. Aim for at least 90 degrees of shoulder turn relative to your hips.

- Trail Foot Positioning: Slightly turn out your trail foot (right foot for right-handed golfers) to allow better hip rotation during the backswing.

- Wrist Position: Keep your lead wrist flat at the top of the backswing. Avoid excessive wrist extension [cupping], as this can open the clubface and lead to slices or fades.

- Backswing Length: While some players benefit from a full backswing, many amateurs gain consistency by shortening their backswing slightly (around three-fourths). This helps maintain control over clubface alignment.

## 3. Initiate Your Downswing Correctly

The transition from backswing to downswing is critical for generating speed and accuracy:

- Hip Rotation First: Start by rotating your hips toward the target before moving your upper body or arms. This sequence creates lag and maximizes power transfer into impact.

- Weight Shift: Transfer weight from your trail foot to your lead foot as you begin swinging down. Avoid hanging back on your trail side, as this can cause thin shots or slices.

- Shallow Angle of Attack: With a driver, aim for an upward angle of attack rather than hitting down on the ball like you would with irons. A shallow approach increases launch angle and reduces spin.

## 4. Impact Position

At impact, several key elements determine whether you'll achieve maximum distance and accuracy:

- Clubhead Behind Hands: Ensure that at impact, your hands are ahead of the clubhead; or at least they should be relatively aligned with it.

- Head Behind Ball: Keep your head positioned behind the ball at impact to encourage an upward strike.

- Square Clubface: The clubface should be square (perpendicular) to both its path and target line at impact.

The Journey Begins

## 5. Follow Through

A proper follow-through ensures that all energy is transferred efficiently into the shot:

- Full Extension: Extend both arms fully after impact while keeping them relaxed. This indicates that you've made solid contact with good energy transfer.

- Balanced Finish Position: End in a balanced position where most of your weight is on your lead foot, facing toward the target.

## Additional Tips for Hitting Off The Tee With a Driver

1. Practice reducing grip pressure if you tend to slice or hook—tight grips often create tension that disrupts smooth swings.

2. Experiment with different tee heights until you find what works best for generating consistent strikes near the sweet spot of your driver face.

3. If you're struggling with consistency, shorten your swing slightly without sacrificing shoulder turn—it's better to have control than extra distance.

By following these steps consistently during practice sessions and rounds, you'll develop better control over trajectory, distance, and accuracy when hitting off the tee with a driver.

# Fairway Woods/Hybrids

## Fairway or Rough

When it comes to longer shots in golf, particularly from the fairway or rough, choosing between fairway woods and hybrids can significantly impact your performance. Both clubs are designed to help golfers achieve distance and accuracy, but their design and functionality cater to different situations. Below is a detailed breakdown of how each club performs in these scenarios.

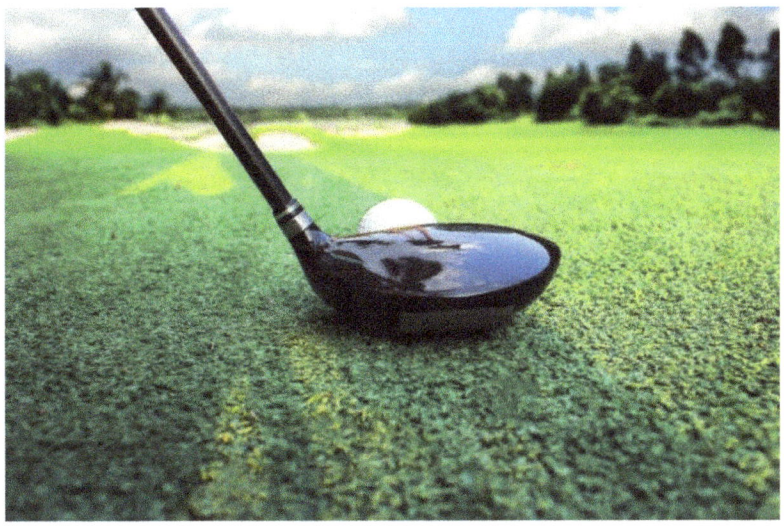

## Fairway Woods for Longer Shot

Fairway woods are specifically designed for long-distance shots, making them an excellent choice when you need to cover significant yardage. Their larger clubheads and lower lofts allow for greater power and distance compared to hybrids or irons. Here's how they perform in various conditions:

**From the Fairway:**

o   Fairway woods, such as the 3-wood or 5-wood, excel on clean lies in the fairway where there is minimal interference with the ball.

o   The larger clubhead provides a higher moment of inertia (MOI), which helps generate more power and stability during the swing.

o   A flatter face with less loft allows for a penetrating ball flight that maximizes roll after landing, making them ideal for reaching greens on par 5s or long par 4s.

o   However, they require precise ball-striking due to their longer shafts and smaller sweet spots compared to hybrids.

**From the Rough:**

o   Fairway woods can be challenging to use from thick rough because their larger clubheads may struggle to cut through dense grass effectively.

o   The low loft of fairway woods makes it harder to get the ball airborne quickly from deep rough, often resulting in reduced carry distance.

**Best Situations for Fairway Woods:**

o   Long approach shots on par 5s or long par 4s.

o   Tee shots on shorter par 4s where accuracy is prioritized over driver distance.

o   Clean lies in light rough or fairways where maximum distance is required.

# Hybrids for Longer Shots

Hybrids are designed as a versatile alternative to both long irons and fairway woods. They combine elements of both club types, offering forgiveness, ease of use, and adaptability across various lies. Here's how they perform:

**From the Fairway:**

o Hybrids are easier to hit than fairway woods due to their shorter shafts and smaller clubheads.

o They have a higher center of gravity (CG) than fairway woods but lower than irons, which helps launch the ball higher with more spin.

o This high launch angle makes hybrids ideal for holding greens on long approach shots since they land with a steeper descent angle compared to fairway woods.

**From the Rough:**

o Hybrids excel in rough conditions because their compact clubhead design allows them to glide through thick grass more easily than fairway woods.

o The rounded sole reduces turf interaction, enabling cleaner contact even from difficult lies.

o Hybrids also provide better control over direction and spin compared to fairway woods when hitting out of trouble areas.

**Best Situations for Hybrids:**

o Long approach shots into greens where precision is critical.

o   Escaping from thick rough or uneven lies where clean contact is difficult with other clubs.

o   Replacing long irons (e.g., 3-iron or 4-iron) for improved consistency and forgiveness.

## Key Differences Between Fairway Woods and Hybrids

| Feature | Fairway Woods | Hybrids |
|---|---|---|
| Clubhead Size | Larger | Smaller |
| Shaft Length | Longer | Shorter |
| Loft Range | Lower (13°–19° typical) | Higher (16°–28° typical) |
| Ball Flight | Lower trajectory with more roll | Higher trajectory with softer landing |
| Forgiveness | Less forgiving | More forgiving |
| Versatility | Best on clean lies | Effective from various lies |

## Which Should You Choose?

The decision between using a fairway wood or hybrid depends largely on your specific situation:

•   If you're hitting off a clean lie in the fairway and need maximum distance, a fairway wood like a 3-wood or 5-wood is likely your best option due to its ability to generate power and roll after landing.

- If you're dealing with thicker rough or an uneven lie—or if you prioritize accuracy over sheer distance—a hybrid will offer better results thanks to its versatility and ease of use.

For most amateur golfers who struggle with consistency using long irons or fairway woods, hybrids are often recommended as they provide a balance between distance, control, and forgiveness.

# Consistency:
# Distance & Accuracy

When it comes to long shots in golf, maintaining both distance and accuracy is a challenge that requires a combination of proper technique, mental focus, and physical conditioning. Below are detailed tips to help you achieve consistency with your long shots:

## 1. Optimize Your Setup for Long Shots

The foundation of any successful golf shot begins with the setup. For long shots, this becomes even more critical as small errors in alignment or posture can magnify over greater distances.

- Ball Position: Place the ball slightly forward in your stance (closer to your lead foot) when using longer clubs like drivers or fairway woods. This allows for an upward strike, maximizing distance.

- Stance Width: Adopt a wider stance for stability during the swing. A wider base helps you maintain balance while generating power.

- Alignment: Ensure your shoulders, hips, and feet are aligned parallel to the target line. Misalignment can cause slices or hooks.

- Grip Pressure: Maintain a light but firm grip on the club. Excessive grip pressure can lead to tension in your arms and shoulders, reducing swing fluidity.

## 2. Focus on Swing Mechanics

Consistency in swing mechanics is essential for achieving both distance and accuracy.

- Smooth Tempo: Avoid swinging too hard in an attempt to gain extra yards. A smooth tempo ensures better control over the clubface at impact.

- Full Shoulder Turn: Rotate your shoulders fully during the backswing while keeping your lower body stable. This creates torque and generates power.

- Weight Transfer: Proper weight transfer is crucial for maximizing energy transfer into the ball. Start with weight balanced between both feet, shift it to your trail leg during the backswing, and then move it back to your lead leg during the downswing.

- Clubface Control: Keep the clubface square throughout the swing by focusing on wrist position. A bowed lead wrist at impact promotes solid contact and reduces side spin.

## 3. Prioritize Timing Over Raw Power

Many golfers mistakenly believe that swinging harder will result in longer shots, but timing plays a far more significant role.

- Release Timing: Release the clubhead at just the right moment to square up the face at impact. Early or late releases can cause hooks or slices.

- Drills for Timing: Practice drills like "hit hard then stop," where you stop your follow-through immediately after impact. This helps develop control over release timing.

## 4. Use Equipment Suited to Your Game

The right equipment can make a significant difference in achieving consistency with long shots.

- Driver Loft: Choose a driver loft that matches your swing speed—higher lofts (10–12 degrees) are better for slower swings, while lower lofts (8–9 degrees) suit faster swings.

- Shaft Flexibility: Ensure that your shaft flex matches your swing speed; too stiff or too flexible shafts can reduce accuracy and distance.

- Ball Selection: Use golf balls designed for distance if you struggle with length off the tee but prioritize those offering low spin rates to improve accuracy.

## 5. Develop Mental Focus

Long shots require not only physical skill but also mental clarity.

- Visualization Techniques: Before hitting a long shot, visualize its trajectory and landing spot clearly in your mind.

- Pre-Shot Routine: Establish a consistent pre-shot routine that includes alignment checks, practice swings, and deep breaths to calm nerves.

- Stay Positive Under Pressure: If you miss-hit a long shot, avoid frustration as it can affect subsequent swings negatively.

## 6. Incorporate Fitness into Your Routine

Physical fitness directly impacts how well you execute long shots.

- Core Strengthening Exercises: A strong core improves rotational power during your swing.

- Flexibility Training: Stretching exercises enhance range of motion in key areas like shoulders, hips, and spine.

- Endurance Workouts: Cardiovascular fitness helps maintain energy levels throughout an 18-hole round.

## 7. Practice Smartly

Practice sessions should be purposeful rather than repetitive.

- Simulate Course Conditions: Practice hitting long shots under conditions similar to those on an actual course (e.g., varying lies or wind).

- Track Performance Metrics: Use launch monitors or GPS devices to measure carry distance, ball speed, spin rate, etc., so you can identify areas needing improvement.

- Focus on Weaknesses: Dedicate extra time to addressing specific issues such as slicing or inconsistent contact.

## Final Thoughts

Consistency with long shots requires attention to detail across multiple aspects of golf—setup, mechanics, timing, equipment selection, mental focus, fitness levels, and practice habits all play vital roles. By systematically addressing each of these areas through focused effort and regular practice sessions tailored toward improvement goals, golfers can significantly enhance their ability to hit long shots accurately while maintaining impressive distances.

# Safety Precautions

Golf is a sport that requires not only skill and precision but also a strong emphasis on safety to ensure the well-being of all players and spectators. Adhering to proper safety precautions is essential, as golf involves swinging clubs at high speeds and hitting balls that can travel at significant velocities. Below are detailed safety measures to follow on the golf course:

## Standing out of Harm's Way when others swing

One of the most critical aspects of golf safety is ensuring you are positioned correctly when another player is taking their shot. This precaution minimizes the risk of being struck by a club or ball.

- **Positioning:** Always stand well away from the player who is about to swing, ideally behind them or off to the side at a safe distance. Never stand directly in front of or in line with their intended shot direction.

- **Peripheral Vision Awareness:** Avoid standing in the player's peripheral vision, as this can be distracting and may cause them to lose focus during their swing.

- **Club Swing Radius:** Be mindful of the club's swing radius, which extends beyond just where the ball lies. Standing too close could result in accidental contact with the club.

## Staying Alert for Errant Shots

Golf balls can travel at speeds exceeding 100 mph, making it crucial to remain vigilant at all times.

- **Listening for Warnings:** Pay attention to shouts of "Fore!"—a universal warning signal indicating an errant shot heading toward people.

- **Quick Reaction:** If you hear "Fore!", immediately cover your head with your arms and crouch down to minimize exposure.

- **Avoid Distractions:** Refrain from using headphones or engaging in activities that reduce your awareness of your surroundings.

## Maintaining Safe Distances

To prevent injuries caused by stray shots or mishandled swings:

- Keep a safe distance (at least several yards) from other players while they are addressing or striking the ball.

- Avoid walking ahead of someone preparing to hit their shot until they have completed it.

- On driving ranges, stay within your designated hitting area and avoid wandering into adjacent lanes.

## Proper Club Handling

Handling golf clubs responsibly reduces risks associated with accidental injuries:

- Never swing a club unless you have checked that no one is within range.

- Avoid practicing full swings outside designated practice areas.

- Carry clubs securely when walking between holes or around crowded areas.

## Awareness Around Carts

Golf carts are convenient but can pose hazards if not used properly:

- Drive cautiously, especially on slopes or near water hazards.

- Ensure passengers are seated before moving the cart.

- Do not drive too close to greens, bunkers, or other players.

## Weather Safety

Weather conditions can create additional risks on the course:

- In case of lightning, seek shelter immediately—do not remain exposed on open fairways or under trees.

- Wear appropriate footwear for wet conditions to avoid slipping on slick surfaces.

## General Etiquette for Safety

Good etiquette often overlaps with safety practices:

- Wait until the group ahead has cleared before taking your shot.

- Avoid rushing others; impatience can lead to mistakes and accidents.

- Respect course rules regarding restricted areas and hazard zones.

By following these guidelines, golfers can enjoy their game while minimizing risks for themselves and others on the course.

# Mental Approach & Strategy

## Staying Positive After Bad Shots

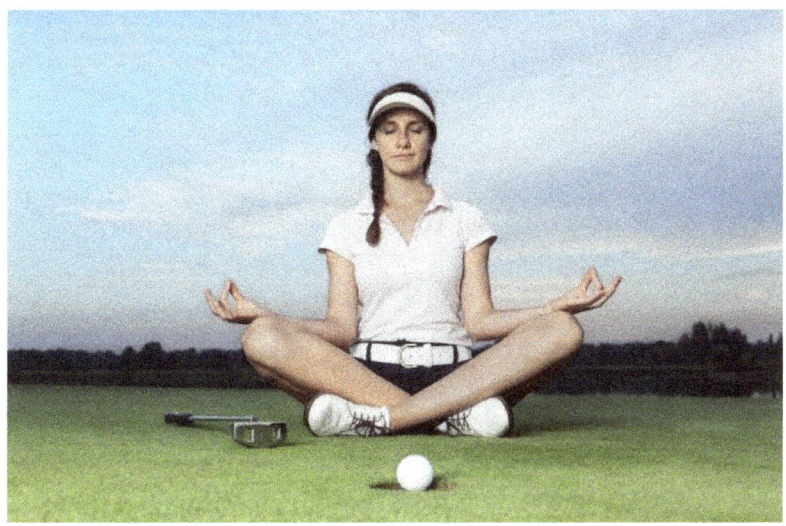

The mental aspect of golf, particularly staying positive after bad shots, is crucial for their development and enjoyment of the game. Golf is a sport where mistakes are inevitable, but how players respond to those mistakes can significantly impact their performance and overall experience. Below is a detailed explanation of strategies to help golfers stay positive after bad shots.

## Reframe How They View Mistakes

The first step to remaining positive is to reframe their perspective on mistakes. Instead of viewing a bad shot as a failure, see it as an opportunity to learn and improve. Even the professional golfers hit bad shots, but what sets them apart is their ability to recover mentally.

- Four possible outcomes of a golf shot:

- o   Good execution with a good result.

- o   Good execution with a bad result.

- o   Bad execution with a good result.

- o   Bad execution with a bad result.

Understand that only focusing on "good execution + good result" will limit their happiness and satisfaction on the course. Celebrate or accept outcomes like "bad execution + good result" or "good execution + bad result" because these still contribute positively to their round.

By broadening what they consider acceptable outcomes, they'll reduce frustration and maintain positivity throughout the game.

**Use Positive Self-Talk**

Positive self-talk is one of the most effective tools for staying optimistic after mistakes. For example:

- Instead of saying, "I'm terrible at this," say, "That wasn't my best shot, but I know I can do better next time."

- Replace "I always mess up this hole" with "I've played this hole well before; I can do it again."

This shift in mindset helps build confidence and keeps players focused on improving rather than dwelling on errors.

**Stay in the Present Moment**

Golf requires focus on each individual shot rather than lingering on past mistakes or worrying about future ones. Learn techniques to stay present:

- Deep breathing exercises before each shot to resets their focus.

- Simple mantras like "One shot at a time" or "Stay calm, stay focused."

- Every new shot presents an opportunity for success.

Staying present prevents negative emotions from snowballing into further mistakes.

**Implement the "Bag-Up Principle"**

A practical way to manage emotions after a bad shot is using physical boundaries like their golf bag as an emotional reset point:

- After hitting a poor shot, allow time (e.g., walking back to their bag) to feel frustrated if necessary.

- Once they reach their bag, then it's time to let go of any lingering negativity and refocus on the next task.

This approach creates a structured way for players to process emotions without letting frustration carry over into subsequent shots.

**Celebrate Small Wins**

Find positives in every round or practice session:

- Highlight small victories such as improved putting accuracy or hitting one great drive.

- Reinforce that progress in golf comes incrementally, so even minor improvements are worth celebrating.

By focusing on achievements rather than setbacks, players will develop resilience and maintain enthusiasm for the game.

## Normalize Mistakes

Making mistakes is part of learning golf—and even professionals make errors regularly during tournaments.

## Practice Visualization Techniques

Visualization can help players prepare mentally for challenging situations:

- Before starting a round or practice session, they can visualize themselves successfully recovering from difficult scenarios (e.g., hitting out of bunkers or recovering from rough terrain).

- This mental preparation builds confidence so they're less likely to feel defeated when faced with adversity during play.

## Focus on Enjoyment Over Perfection

Intrinsic motivations like enjoying time outdoors or spending quality moments with friends/family over extrinsic goals like achieving perfect scores. When players prioritize enjoyment over perfectionism, they're more likely to stay positive regardless of performance fluctuations.

## Set Realistic Expectations

Players should set achievable goals tailored to their current skill level rather than comparing themselves unfairly to others (especially experienced golfers). For instance:

- A goal could be reducing three-putts instead of expecting flawless putting.

- Another goal might be simply keeping composure after every hole regardless of score.

Realistic expectations reduce pressure while fostering steady improvement over time.

**Constructive Feedback After Rounds**

After finishing a round or practice session, think about both successes and areas for improvement in an encouraging manner:

- Start by highlighting what went well ("My drives were much straighter today!").

- Then address challenges constructively ("I'll work on bunker shots next practice.").

This balanced feedback reinforces progress while framing setbacks as opportunities for growth rather than failures.

By introducing these strategies early in their golfing journey, golfers will develop strong mental habits that not only improve performance but also enhance their overall enjoyment of the game. Staying positive after bad shots becomes second nature when players learn how to reframe mistakes, use positive self-talk, remain present-focused, celebrate small wins, normalize errors, visualize success, prioritize fun over perfectionism, set realistic goals, and receive constructive feedback regularly.

# Setting Goals for Improvement

Setting realistic goals is a cornerstone of improving your mental approach and overall strategy in golf. This process involves creating clear, measurable, and achievable objectives that guide your practice sessions and on-course performance. By focusing on specific areas for improvement, you can maintain motivation, track progress, and build confidence over time. Let's break this down step by step:

## Why Setting Realistic Goals Matters

1. Focuses Your Efforts: Golf is a complex game with numerous skills to master, from driving accuracy to putting precision. Without clear goals, it's easy to spread your efforts too thin or practice without purpose. Realistic goals help you concentrate on the most critical aspects of your game.

2. Builds Confidence: Achieving smaller, attainable milestones reinforces a sense of accomplishment. This positive reinforcement boosts confidence and encourages continued improvement.

3. Reduces Frustration: Unrealistic expectations can lead to disappointment and frustration when progress doesn't come as quickly as hoped. Realistic goals ensure that you set yourself up for success rather than failure.

## How to Set Realistic Goals

1. Assess Your Current Skill Level: Start by evaluating where you stand in terms of your golf abilities. Use metrics like handicap, driving accuracy percentage, greens in regulation (GIR), or average putts per round to identify strengths and weaknesses.

o For example, if your current driving accuracy is 50%, a realistic goal might be to improve it to 60% over the next three months.

2. Make Goals Specific and Measurable: Vague goals like "I want to get better at golf" are hard to achieve because they lack focus. Instead, set precise targets such as:

o Reducing your handicap by two strokes within six months.

o Hitting at least 70% of fairways during a round.

o Improving putting consistency by sinking 80% of putts within five feet.

3. Set Short-Term and Long-Term Goals: Break down larger objectives into smaller steps that can be achieved over weeks or months.

o Short-term goal: Practice bunker shots three times a week for one month.

o Long-term goal: Improve sand save percentage from 30% to 50% within six months.

4. Ensure Goals Are Achievable Yet Challenging: While it's important not to set the bar too high, goals should still push you out of your comfort zone enough to encourage growth.

## Examples of Realistic Golf Goals

• Lowering your handicap by one stroke every three months through focused practice on weak areas such as short game or approach shots.

• Increasing greens in regulation (GIR) from 40% to 50% over the course of a season by working on mid-iron accuracy during practice sessions.

- Reducing three-putts per round from an average of four to two by dedicating extra time each week to lag putting drills.

## The Role of Goal Setting in Mental Approach

1. Improves Focus During Rounds: When you have specific goals in mind, it becomes easier to stay mentally engaged throughout an entire round instead of dwelling on past mistakes or worrying about future holes.

2. Encourages Positive Thinking: Achieving small victories along the way helps reinforce optimism and resilience—key components of a strong mental game in golf.

3. Provides Motivation for Practice: Knowing exactly what you're working toward makes practice sessions more productive and enjoyable.

## Tracking Progress

To ensure that you're making strides toward achieving your goals:

- Keep detailed records of performance metrics during rounds (e.g., fairways hit, GIRs, number of putts).

- Reflect regularly on what's working well and what needs adjustment in both practice routines and mental strategies.

By setting realistic goals tailored specifically to your current skill level and aspirations, you create a structured pathway for continuous improvement while maintaining a positive mindset throughout the journey.

## Learning Course Management Strategies

Golf is as much a mental game as it is a physical one, and mastering course management strategies can significantly improve your performance. The ability to decide when to play aggressively versus conservatively is a critical skill that separates good golfers from great ones. Below is a detailed breakdown of how to approach this aspect of the game step by step.

# Self-Assessment

## Understanding Strengths and Weaknesses

The foundation of effective course management begins with an honest evaluation of your own abilities. Ask yourself:

- Are you better at long drives or accurate tee shots?

- Is your short game reliable, or do you struggle with putting under pressure?

- Do you have consistent control over shot shapes (e.g., fades, draws)?

Knowing your strengths allows you to lean into them during high-risk situations, while understanding your weaknesses helps you avoid unnecessary mistakes. For example:

- If you're not confident in hitting long irons, it might be better to lay up on a par 5 rather than attempting to reach the green in two.

- If accuracy off the tee is your strength, focus on positioning rather than distance.

## Evaluating Each Hole: Risk vs. Reward

Every hole on a golf course presents unique challenges and opportunities. To decide whether to play aggressively or conservatively, consider the following factors:

### Tee Shots

- **Aggressive Play:** Choose this approach if the fairway is wide and hazards are minimal. For example, hitting a driver on a par 4 with no significant trouble can set up an easier approach shot.

- **Conservative Play:** Opt for this when hazards like bunkers, water, or out-of-bounds areas are present near your landing zone. A shorter club like a hybrid or iron may keep you safely in play.

**Approach Shots**

- **Aggressive Play:** Go for the pin if it's accessible (e.g., located in the center of the green) and there's little risk of missing badly.

- **Conservative Play:** Aim for the middle of the green when pins are tucked near hazards ("sucker pins"). This minimizes risk while still giving you a chance at par or birdie.

**Short Game Decisions**

When chipping or pitching around the green:

- Be aggressive only if you have confidence in your ability to execute high-risk shots (e.g., flop shots over bunkers).

- Otherwise, prioritize leaving yourself an uphill putt rather than risking leaving it short or in trouble.

## Key Factors Influencing Aggression vs. Conservatism

Several variables should guide your decision-making process:

**Course Layout**

Analyze each hole's design:

- Wide-open fairways and greens encourage more aggressive play.

- Narrow fairways with penalizing roughs demand conservative strategies.

## Hazards

Identify all potential trouble spots such as water hazards, bunkers, and out-of-bounds areas:

- Avoid aiming directly at pins located near these hazards unless absolutely necessary.

## Weather Conditions

Windy conditions often necessitate conservative play:

- Strong headwinds make aggressive shots harder to control.

- Tailwinds may allow for longer carries but increase unpredictability.

## Your Current Performance

Adjust based on how you're playing that day:

- If you're striking the ball well and feeling confident, take calculated risks.

- If you're struggling with consistency, focus on minimizing errors by playing conservatively.

## Creating a Hole-by-Hole Game Plan

Before starting your round, map out each hole strategically

1. Identify safe landing zones for tee shots.

2. Decide which holes offer scoring opportunities (e.g., reachable par 5s) versus those where par is an acceptable outcome.

3. Plan lay-up distances that leave comfortable yardages for approach shots.

For example: On a par 4 with water guarding one side of the green and no bailout area nearby:

- A conservative strategy would involve aiming for the center of the fairway off the tee and then targeting the middle of the green on your approach shot.

**Staying Flexible During Your Round**

While having a pre-round strategy is essential, adaptability is equally important during play:

1. Adjust based on changing conditions such as wind direction or firmness of greens.

2. Factor in how you're performing—if you've hit several poor drives early on, consider scaling back aggression until confidence returns.

**Mental Discipline: Managing Emotions Under Pressure**

Effective course management requires staying calm and focused throughout your round:

1. Avoid chasing birdies unnecessarily after making bogeys; instead, stick to your plan.

2. Accept that not every hole will be an opportunity to score—sometimes playing for bogey instead of double bogey can save strokes over 18 holes.

## Post-Round Reflection: Learning From Experience

After completing your round:

1. Review decisions made during key moments—did aggressive plays pay off? Were conservative choices too cautious?

2. Keep notes about specific holes where adjustments could improve future performance (e.g., aiming further right off certain tees).

By consistently reflecting on past rounds and refining strategies accordingly, you'll develop better instincts for managing courses effectively.

# Practice Tips & Drills

## Creating a Practice Routine That Balances Driving Range Time with Short Game Practice

To create an effective golf practice routine that balances driving range time with short game practice, it's essential to focus on structured, purposeful sessions. The goal is to allocate time efficiently between the long game (driving range) and the short game (shots within 100 yards, chipping, pitching, bunker play, and putting). Below is a detailed step-by-step guide:

### Step 1: Assess Your Current Skill Level

Before creating a balanced routine, evaluate your strengths and weaknesses. For example:

- If you struggle with accuracy off the tee or distance control with irons, prioritize more driving range time.

- If you lose strokes around the greens or in bunkers, dedicate more time to short game practice.

A general rule of thumb for most golfers is to spend **60% of your practice time on the short game** and **40% on full-swing practice**, as the majority of strokes in a round occur within 100 yards.

### Step 2: Structure Your Weekly Practice Schedule

Divide your available weekly practice hours into specific sessions for both driving range work and short game drills. Here's an example schedule for someone practicing 3 times per week:

## Day 1: Driving Range Focus (60 minutes)

- **Warm-Up (10 minutes):** Stretch and hit 15-20 wedge shots at half-swing to loosen up.

- **Full Swing Practice (40 minutes):**

    o   Work on driver accuracy by hitting 10 balls at specific fairway targets.

    o   Hit mid-irons (7-iron through pitching wedge) focusing on ball flight and trajectory control.

    o   Finish with long irons or hybrids for distance consistency.

- **Short Game Integration (10 minutes):** End by hitting pitch shots from 30–50 yards to simulate approach shots.

## Day 2: Short Game Focus (60 minutes)

- **Warm-Up (5 minutes):** Stretch and take light swings with wedges.

- **Chipping & Pitching Drills (20 minutes):**

    o   Practice bump-and-run shots using an 8-iron or pitching wedge.

    o   Work on high lofted pitches from rough or tight lies using a sand wedge or lob wedge.

    o   Aim for landing zones within a small circle around the pin.

- **Bunker Play (15 minutes):**

    o   Hit sand shots focusing on open clubface technique and consistent contact.

- o Try different distances by varying swing length while maintaining proper form.

- **Putting Practice (20 minutes):**

  - o Start with lag putts from 20–40 feet to improve distance control.

  - o Finish with shorter putts inside six feet to build confidence under pressure.

## Day 3: Balanced Session (90 minutes)

Split this session evenly between driving range work and short game drills:

1. Spend the first half working on full swings at the range:

   - o Alternate between drivers, irons, hybrids, and wedges every few shots to simulate course conditions.

   - o Use alignment sticks or markers for target-focused practice.

2. Dedicate the second half entirely to short game:

   - o Combine chipping drills with putting drills into simulated "up-and-down" challenges where you chip onto the green and then putt out.

## Step 3. Incorporate Specific Drills for Both Areas

To maximize improvement during each session, use targeted drills:

## Driving Range Drills

1. **Fairway Finder Drill:** Use your driver or fairway wood to hit balls into a narrow target area simulating a fairway width. This

improves accuracy off the tee.

2. **Distance Ladder Drill:** Hit three consecutive shots increasing in distance but maintaining control—e.g., start with a pitching wedge at 100 yards, then move up to an 8-iron at 140 yards, followed by a hybrid at 180 yards.

**Short Game Drills**

1. **Circle Drill for Putting:** Place five balls in a circle around the hole at three-foot intervals. Putt each ball until all are holed out without missing consecutively, this builds confidence in close-range putts.

2. **Landing Zone Drill:** Place towels or markers at various distances on the green (e.g., 10, 20, and 30 yards). Chip balls aiming for these zones before rolling them toward pins.

**Step 4: Track Progress Over Time**

Keep notes after each session about what worked well and what needs improvement:

- Record how many fairways you hit during driving range sessions or how many chips landed within six feet of the hole during short game practice.

- Adjust your routine based on these observations—for instance, if bunker play remains weak despite dedicated time, increase focus there.

**Step 5: Balance Practice With On-Course Play**

While structured practice is critical, playing actual rounds helps translate skills into real-world scenarios:

1. During rounds, identify areas where strokes are lost most frequently—this feedback should guide future practice priorities.

2. Simulate course-like conditions during practice by alternating between full swings and short-game shots instead of isolating them entirely.

## Summary of Time Allocation Per Session

For most golfers practicing two hours per week:

1. Warm-up: ~10% of total time

2. Driving Range/Full Swing Work: ~40%

3. Short Game Practice (~50%):

   o Chipping/Pitching/Bunker Shots (~30%)

   o Putting (~20%)

Adjust these percentages based on personal weaknesses—players struggling off the tee may need closer to equal balance between driving range work and short game focus.

# Drills for Juniors

Improving coordination in junior golfers is essential for their development, but it's equally important to keep the drills fun and engaging so they stay motivated. Below are several actionable and enjoyable drills designed specifically for juniors to enhance their hand-eye coordination, balance, and overall athleticism while ensuring they have a great time.

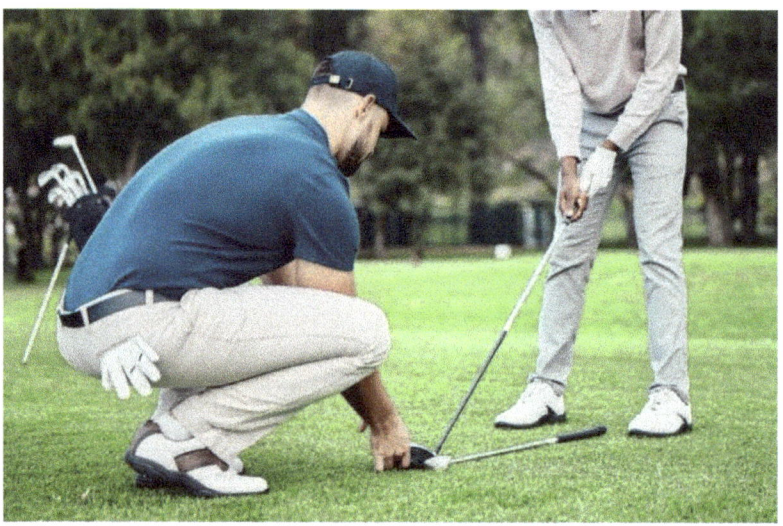

## 1. Ball Toss and Catch with a Golf Club

This drill helps juniors develop hand-eye coordination and get comfortable handling a golf club.

- How to Perform:

    o Have the junior hold a wedge or short iron in one hand.

    o Place a soft foam or plastic ball on the ground.

- o Instruct them to scoop the ball up using the clubface and toss it gently into the air.

- o They should then try to catch the ball with their free hand.

- o Alternate hands holding the club after every few attempts.

- Why It Works: This drill improves control of the clubface, enhances focus, and strengthens both dominant and non-dominant hands.

- Make It Fun: Turn it into a game by challenging them to see how many successful tosses and catches they can do in a row without dropping the ball.

## 2. Clubface Balancing Drill

This activity builds awareness of the clubhead position while improving fine motor skills.

- How to Perform:

  - o Give the junior golfer a wedge or putter.

  - o Place a small foam or plastic ball on the clubface.

  - o Ask them to balance the ball on the face of the club for as long as possible without letting it fall off.

  - o Once they master this, challenge them to walk around while balancing the ball on their clubface.

- Why It Works: This drill develops steady hands, concentration, and an understanding of how subtle movements affect balance.

- Make It Fun: Create an obstacle course where they must navigate through cones or other objects while keeping the ball balanced on their clubface.

## 3. Bounce-and-Catch Challenge

This drill focuses on timing, rhythm, and precision with both hands.

- How to Perform:

    o Using a wedge or short iron, have juniors bounce a foam or plastic ball off the clubface repeatedly without letting it drop.

    o Start with one hand (dominant), then switch to their non-dominant hand.

    o For added difficulty, challenge them to alternate hands after every bounce or flip the club between bounces (360-degree flip).

- Why It Works: This improves hand-eye coordination, grip control, and adaptability when handling different shots during play.

- Make It Fun: Set goals like achieving five consecutive bounces or competing against friends/siblings for who can achieve more bounces in one minute.

## 4. Target Practice with Soft Balls

This drill introduces accuracy while keeping things playful indoors or outdoors.

- How to Perform:

    o Set up targets such as buckets, hula hoops, or small nets at varying distances from where they stand.

- o Provide soft foam balls that won't damage surroundings if played indoors.

- o Have juniors chip balls toward these targets using wedges or even putters for closer distances.

- Why It Works: This builds spatial awareness, distance control, and precision—all critical skills for golf success.

- Make It Fun: Award points based on which target is hit (e.g., closer targets = fewer points; farther ones = more points). Turn it into a friendly competition among peers or family members!

## 5. Balance Beam Putting Drill

Balance is crucial in golf swings; this drill makes learning balance fun while incorporating putting skills.

- How to Perform:

- o Lay down a narrow piece of wood (or use painter's tape) as an imaginary balance beam on flat ground.

- o Have juniors stand on this "beam" while attempting short putts toward a target like a cup or small hole cut out of cardboard.

- Why It Works: This teaches weight distribution during putting strokes while improving stability and focus under pressure.

- Make It Fun: Add challenges like standing on one foot while putting or increasing distance from the target over time. Reward successful attempts with small prizes!

## 6. Balloon Golf Game

A lighthearted game that emphasizes swing control without worrying about hitting hard objects.

- How to Perform:

    o Blow up several balloons and scatter them across an open area (indoors works too).

    o Give each junior golfer a lightweight plastic golf club (or even just their hands mimicking swings).

    o The goal is to "hit" balloons toward designated zones marked by cones or tape lines on the floor/ground.

- Why It Works: This helps juniors practice controlled swings without fear of missing shots. The light resistance of balloons also encourages proper follow-through motions.

- Make It Fun: Time how quickly they can move all balloons into specific zones—or let them compete against others in balloon races!

## 7. Ladder Drill for Footwork Coordination

Although not directly involving clubs, this drill enhances footwork— a key component of good golf posture and swing mechanics.

- How to Perform:

    o Lay down an agility ladder (or create one using chalk/tape) on flat ground.

    o Have juniors perform various footwork patterns through each rung:

- Two feet in each square

- One-foot hops

- Side shuffles

- Backward steps

- After completing each pattern through the ladder, have them take practice swings focusing on maintaining balance throughout their motion.

- Why It Works: Good footwork translates into better weight transfer during swings and improved overall athleticism necessary for golf performance.

- Make It Fun: Incorporate music beats so they step along rhythmically—or race against friends/family members through different patterns!

## Top Tips for Keeping Juniors Engaged:

1. Use bright-colored equipment like foam balls or cones—they're visually appealing!

2. Keep sessions short but dynamic—15–20 minutes per activity works best for younger kids' attention spans.

3. Offer rewards like stickers or small prizes for completing challenges successfully—it boosts motivation!

4. Encourage creativity—let kids invent new games using clubs/balls within safe boundaries!

By combining these drills with positive reinforcement and fun competition elements, you'll ensure that juniors not only improve their coordination but also develop lasting enthusiasm for golf.

The Journey Begins

# Putting Practice is Essential

It Accounts for Many Strokes in a Round

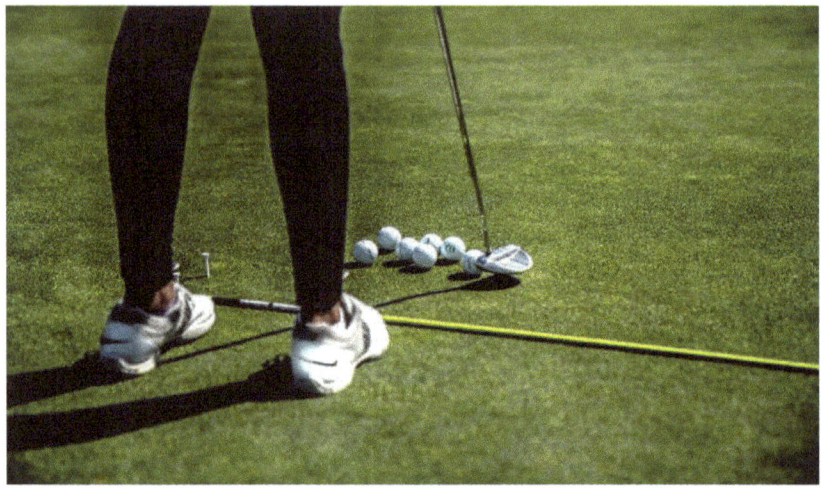

Putting is one of the most critical aspects of golf, as it directly impacts your score more than almost any other part of the game. On average, putting accounts for approximately 40% of all strokes during a round, making it an area where players can significantly improve their performance and lower their scores with focused practice. Below is a detailed breakdown of why practicing putting is essential and actionable advice to help you refine this skill.

## Why Putting Practice Is Crucial

### High Percentage of Total Strokes

In an average round, golfers take about 30-36 putts out of the total 70-100 strokes they play. This means that nearly half your game happens on the green. Improving your putting efficiency can lead to immediate reductions in your overall score without requiring changes to other parts of your game like driving or approach shots.

## Short Putts Are Key Scoring Opportunities

Professional golfers make over 90% of putts within five feet, while amateurs often struggle with these short but crucial opportunities. Missing short putts adds unnecessary strokes to your scorecard, which can be avoided with consistent practice.

## Lag Putting Reduces Three-Putts

Long-distance putting (lag putting) is another critical skill that prevents three-putting on greens. The ability to control distance and leave the ball close to the hole from long range ensures fewer wasted strokes.

## Pressure Situations Demand Confidence

Tournament play or high-pressure rounds often come down to clutch putts on the green. Practicing putting builds confidence in these situations, helping you sink critical putts when it matters most.

## Strokes Gained Putting Statistic

On professional tours, "strokes gained putting" measures how much better a player performs on the greens compared to their peers. Even small improvements in putting can lead to significant competitive advantages.

# Actionable Advice for Practicing Putting

## Develop a Consistent Routine

o   Create a pre-putt routine that includes alignment, visualization, and focus on your target line.

o   Stick to this routine during practice and rounds so it becomes second nature under pressure.

## Practice Short Putts Regularly

o   Dedicate time specifically to putts within five feet since these are high-percentage scoring opportunities.

o   Use drills like the "clock drill," where you place balls around the hole at equal distances (e.g., three feet) and work on sinking each one consecutively.

## Work on Distance Control for Lag Putting

o   Practice hitting putts from varying distances (20-50 feet) with the goal of leaving them within a three-foot radius around the hole.

o   Use alignment aids or tees placed around the hole as targets for lag-putting drills.

## Focus on Green Reading Skills

o   Learn how to assess slopes and breaks by walking around the hole and observing from different angles.

o   Use tools like AimPoint Express or similar techniques to improve accuracy in reading greens.

## Use Feedback Tools During Practice

o   Incorporate training aids like alignment sticks, putting mirrors, or laser guides to ensure proper setup and stroke mechanics.

o   Record yourself practicing so you can analyze your stroke consistency and make adjustments as needed.

**Simulate Pressure Situations**

o Add pressure by setting goals during practice sessions (e.g., make 10 consecutive three-footers before moving on).

o Play games against yourself or others where missed putts have consequences (like restarting a drill).

**Track Your Progress Over Time**

o Keep statistics during rounds such as total putts per round, percentage made from specific distances, and number of three-putts.

o Review these stats regularly to identify areas needing improvement and adjust your practice accordingly.

**Balance Mechanics With Feel Practice**

o While technical drills are important, also spend time practicing feel-based exercises like closing your eyes while stroking short putts or focusing only on tempo rather than mechanics.

**Dedicate Time Solely for Putting Practice**

o Set aside at least 30 minutes per practice session exclusively for putting drills.

o Divide this time between short putts, lag putting, green reading exercises, and pressure simulations.

**Play Games That Mimic Real Scenarios**

o Engage in games like "21" (where you try to get as close as possible without going over par) or "Around-the-World" drills that simulate real-course challenges while keeping practice fun and engaging.

## Benefits You Can Expect From Focused Putting Practice

- Fewer three-putt holes due to improved lag putting skills.

- Higher conversion rates on short putts leading directly to lower scores.

- Increased confidence under pressure during competitive rounds.

- Better understanding of green reading resulting in more accurate lines.

- Overall reduction in total strokes per round by improving efficiency on the greens.

By dedicating consistent effort toward improving your putting through structured practice routines and targeted drills, you can shave multiple strokes off your game without needing significant changes elsewhere in your playstyle.

# Prepping for Your First Round

## Booking Tee Times at Courses

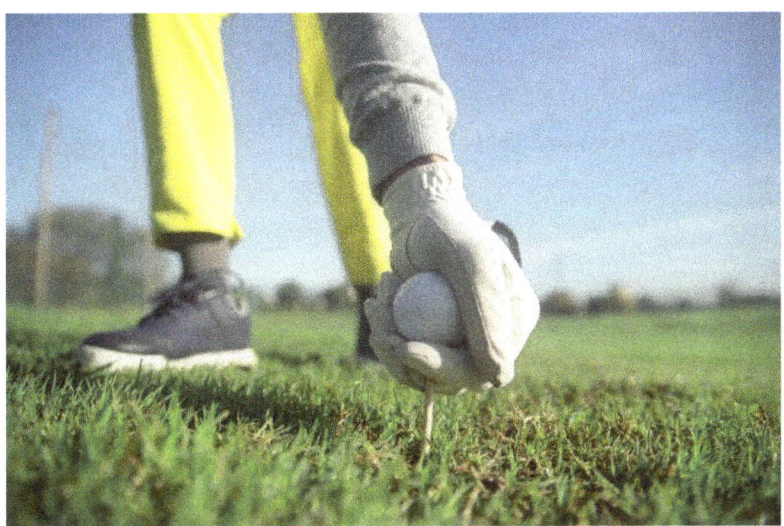

When preparing to play your first full round of golf, booking a tee time is an essential step. For beginners and juniors, it's important to choose courses and times that will make the experience enjoyable and stress-free. Here's a detailed guide on how to approach this process:

### 1. Understand What a Tee Time Is

A tee time is the specific time you are scheduled to begin your round of golf. Think of it as a reservation at a restaurant—it ensures you have a spot on the course at a designated time. Without booking one, especially during busy periods, you risk not being able to play.

### 2. Choose Beginner-Friendly Golf Courses

Not all courses are equally suited for beginners or juniors. Look for courses that meet the following criteria:

- Shorter Yardages: Opt for courses with shorter total distances (4,000–5,500 yards from the forward tees). These are less intimidating and more manageable for new players.

- Beginner-Friendly Reviews: Many online platforms allow golfers to filter reviews by skill level. Look for reviews from players with higher handicaps (20+), as these often highlight beginner-friendly experiences.

- Public or Municipal Courses: Public courses tend to be more welcoming and relaxed compared to private clubs, which may have stricter rules or expectations.

- Junior Programs: Some courses specifically cater to juniors with special programs, discounted rates, or shorter "junior tees."

## 3. Book During Off-Peak Hours

Beginners and juniors should aim to play when the course is less crowded to reduce pressure and allow more time per shot. Consider these options:

- Twilight Hours: Late afternoon or early evening rounds are typically quieter and often come with discounted rates.

- Midweek Play: If schedules allow, playing during weekdays (especially mid-afternoon) can help avoid weekend crowds.

- Check Online Tee Sheets: Many courses now display their availability online through their websites or platforms like GolfNow. This allows you to identify less busy times before booking.

## 4. How to Book Your Tee Time

There are several ways to reserve your spot:

- Online Booking Systems: Most modern golf courses offer online reservations either directly through their website or via third-party platforms like GolfNow or TeeOff.

- Call the Pro Shop: If online booking isn't available or if you have questions about beginner-friendliness, call the course directly. The staff can recommend suitable times and provide guidance on what to expect.

- Walk-Up Option (Risky): While some public courses accept walk-ups without reservations, this is not recommended unless you're certain the course won't be busy.

## 5. Confirm Course Policies

Before finalizing your booking, check these details:

- Rental Clubs Availability: If you don't own clubs yet, confirm whether rentals are available and reserve them in advance if needed.

- Dress Code Requirements: Some courses have specific dress codes; ensure you adhere by wearing appropriate attire such as collared shirts and golf shoes.

- Cancellation Policy: Understand the course's cancellation policy in case plans change.

## 6. Prepare for Your First Round

Once your tee time is booked:

- Arrive at least 30 minutes early so you can check in at the pro shop, warm up on the practice range or putting green, and get comfortable with your surroundings.

- Bring essentials like balls, tees, gloves, water bottles, snacks, sunscreen, and cash for tips if needed.

By carefully selecting beginner-friendly courses during off-peak hours and ensuring all logistics are handled beforehand, new golfers can focus on enjoying their first full round without unnecessary stress.

# First Full Round of Golf

Playing your first full round of golf can be an exciting yet slightly overwhelming experience. Preparation is key to ensuring you enjoy the game and avoid unnecessary stress. Below is a detailed guide on what beginners need to know before stepping onto the course, focusing specifically on what to bring, including essential items like water bottles, snacks, and sunscreen.

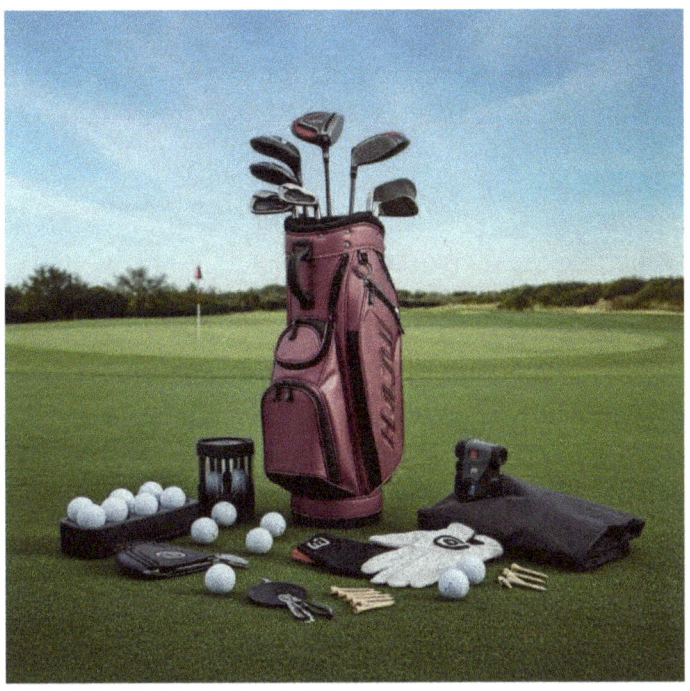

## 1. Essential Items for Hydration and Nutrition

Golf rounds typically last 4-5 hours, and during this time, you'll be walking or riding across the course under varying weather conditions. Staying hydrated and energized is critical for maintaining focus and stamina throughout the game.

The Journey Begins

- Water Bottle: Always carry a reusable water bottle or two filled with water or an electrolyte drink. Dehydration can affect your performance and overall health, especially if you're playing in warm weather.

- Snacks: Pack light, energy-boosting snacks such as granola bars, trail mix, fruit (like bananas or apples), or protein bars. These are easy to eat between holes without disrupting your game. Avoid heavy meals that might make you sluggish.

## 2. Sun Protection

Golf courses are open spaces with minimal shade, so protecting yourself from sun exposure is crucial.

- Sunscreen: Apply sunscreen with at least SPF 30 before starting your round and reapply every two hours if you're out in the sun for extended periods. Choose a sweat-resistant formula for better durability.

- Hat/Cap: A wide-brimmed hat or baseball cap will shield your face from direct sunlight.

- Sunglasses: Polarized sunglasses help reduce glare from the sun and improve visibility when tracking your ball.

## 3. Comfort Accessories

Comfortable gear ensures you stay focused on your game rather than distractions caused by discomfort.

- Towel: A small towel is useful for wiping sweat off your hands or cleaning dirt off clubs and balls.

- Gloves: Golf gloves provide grip stability while preventing blisters during swings.

- Band-Aids/First Aid Kit: Minor injuries like blisters or scrapes can occur; having Band-Aids or a small first aid kit is helpful.

## 4. Weather Preparedness

Weather conditions can change quickly during a round of golf.

- Rain Gear: Bring a lightweight rain jacket or umbrella in case of unexpected rain showers.

- Extra Clothing Layers: If it's chilly in the morning but expected to warm up later, dress in layers that you can easily remove as needed.

## 5. Miscellaneous Items

These additional items will make your first round more enjoyable:

- Mobile Phone (on Silent): For emergencies or using GPS apps to navigate the course layout.

- Ball Marker & Tees: Essential tools for marking your ball's position on the green and setting up shots at the tee box.

- Extra Golf Balls: As a beginner, losing balls is common—carry extras so you don't run out mid-round.

## What You Need To Know Before Your First Round

### 1. Understanding the Basics of Keeping Score

Before playing your first full round of golf, it's important to understand how scoring works. Golf is typically played in one of two formats: stroke play or match play, but for beginners, stroke play is the most common and straightforward format. Here's a breakdown:

- Stroke Play Scoring: In stroke play, every shot you take counts as one stroke. The goal is to complete each hole in as few strokes as possible. At the end of the round (usually 18 holes), you add up all your strokes for a total score.

  - Each hole has a "par," which is the expected number of strokes it should take to complete that hole (e.g., par 3, par 4, or par 5). If you finish a hole in fewer strokes than par, that's great! If it takes more strokes than par, don't worry—this is common for beginners.

  - For example:

    - A score of 3 on a par-3 hole = Par

    - A score of 4 on a par-3 hole = Bogey (+1)

    - A score of 2 on a par-3 hole = Birdie (-1)

- Honesty in Scoring: Golf relies heavily on personal integrity because players are responsible for keeping their own scores. After each hole, write down your total strokes on your scorecard. If you're unsure about a rule or how many strokes to count (e.g., penalties), ask someone in your group for clarification.

## 2. Focusing on Fun Over Competition

As a beginner, it's crucial to prioritize enjoyment over competition during your first rounds. Here are some tips to help you focus on having fun:

- Don't Worry About Your Score Too Much: While keeping an honest score is part of golf etiquette, don't stress about achieving low scores right away. It's normal for beginners to have high scores and make mistakes—it's all part of learning.

  o Instead of obsessing over every shot, celebrate small victories like hitting the ball solidly off the tee or sinking a long putt.

  o Consider using "beginner-friendly" rules such as allowing yourself extra attempts off the tee (a "mulligan") or picking up your ball after reaching double-par (e.g., six shots on a par-3).

- Play at Your Own Pace: Golf can be intimidating when playing with experienced golfers who may move faster or hit better shots. Don't feel pressured—play at a pace that feels comfortable while being mindful not to hold up other groups behind you.

  o If you're struggling on a particular hole, pick up your ball and move on to keep things moving.

- Enjoy the Social Aspect: Golf isn't just about hitting great shots; it's also about spending time outdoors and enjoying good company. Use this opportunity to bond with friends or meet new people.

## 3. Beginner-Friendly Tips for Scoring and Rules

To make scoring easier and reduce frustration during your first rounds:

- Use Handicap-Friendly Formats: Many courses offer handicap systems that adjust scores based on skill level. This can level the playing field if you're golfing with more experienced players.

The Journey Begins

- Learn Basic Penalty Rules Gradually:

  o Add one penalty stroke if you hit out-of-bounds or into water hazards.

  o Drop your ball near where it went out-of-bounds instead of returning to the original spot (to save time).

- Practice Gimme Putts: To speed up play and reduce frustration, agree with your group that very short putts (within two feet) can be considered "gimmes," meaning they're automatically counted as made without actually putting them.

By focusing less on competition and more on learning and having fun, you'll build confidence and develop skills naturally over time.

# Fitness

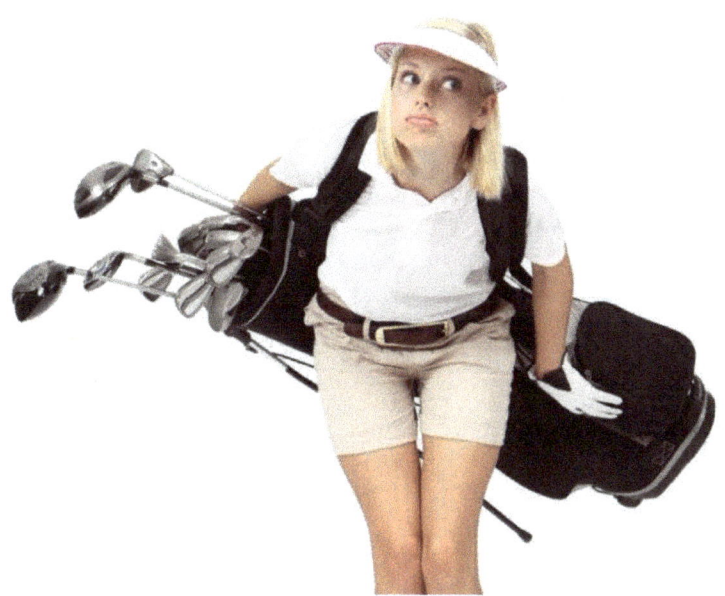

Golf is often perceived as a leisurely sport, but it requires a surprising amount of physical fitness to play effectively and avoid injury. For beginner golfers and weekend players, incorporating a fitness routine tailored to the demands of golf can significantly improve performance, consistency, and overall enjoyment on the course. This chapter will guide you through the essential components of a golf-specific fitness program designed for beginners and casual players.

## Why Fitness Matters for Golfers

Golf involves repetitive movements that require flexibility, strength, balance, endurance, and mental focus. A well-rounded fitness program not only enhances your swing mechanics but also reduces the risk of injuries such as lower back pain or shoulder strain. For weekend players who may not have time for extensive training sessions, focusing on key areas can yield noticeable improvements in both your game and overall health.

## Key Areas of Focus

To build an effective fitness program for beginner golfers and weekend players, prioritize these five areas:

### 1. Flexibility and Mobility

Flexibility is critical in golf because it allows you to achieve a full range of motion during your swing. Mobility ensures that your joints move freely without restriction.

- **Dynamic Stretches (Pre-Round):** Perform leg swings, arm circles, torso twists, or inchworms before playing to loosen up muscles.

- **Static Stretches (Post-Round):** After playing or practicing, use stretches like hamstring stretches, quad stretches, seated spinal twists, or hip flexor stretches to maintain flexibility over time.

- **Target Areas:** Focus on hips (critical for rotation), shoulders (for arm movement), spine (for twisting), and wrists (for grip).

### 2. Core Strength

Your core is the powerhouse of your golf swing. A strong core provides stability during rotation and helps generate power while maintaining control.

- **Beginner Exercises:**
  - Planks: Hold a plank position for 20–30 seconds initially; gradually increase duration as you progress.

o Russian Twists: Sit on the floor with feet off the ground; twist your torso side-to-side while holding a light weight or medicine ball.

o Deadbugs: Lie on your back with arms extended toward the ceiling; alternate lowering opposite arms and legs while keeping your core engaged.

## 3. Balance and Stability

Balance is essential for maintaining proper posture throughout your swing. Stability ensures you can transfer energy efficiently from your lower body to upper body.

- **Beginner Exercises:**

  o Single-Leg Balance: Stand on one leg for 20–30 seconds; switch legs. To increase difficulty, close your eyes or stand on an unstable surface like a foam pad.

  o Lunges: Perform forward lunges with controlled movements to strengthen legs while improving balance.

  o Side Plank Variations: Build lateral stability by holding side planks for short durations.

## 4. Strength Training

Strength training improves muscle endurance and helps prevent injuries by reinforcing key muscle groups used in golf.

- **Focus Areas:** Prioritize functional exercises that mimic golf movements:

  o Deadlifts (with light weights): Strengthen hamstrings, glutes, and lower back.

- o Kettlebell Swings: Improve hip mobility while building explosive power.

- o Dumbbell Rows: Target upper back muscles critical for maintaining posture during swings.

For beginners or those new to strength training, start with bodyweight exercises like squats or push-ups before progressing to weights.

**5. Cardiovascular Fitness**

While golf may not seem physically taxing at first glance, walking long distances across uneven terrain requires stamina—especially if you're carrying your bag.

- **Beginner Cardio Options:**

  - o Walking briskly around the course instead of using a cart is an excellent way to build endurance naturally.

  - o Incorporate low-impact cardio activities like cycling or swimming into your weekly routine to improve heart health without straining joints.

Aim for at least 20–30 minutes of moderate-intensity cardio three times per week.

## How to Structure Your Golf Fitness Routine

For beginner golfers who may only have limited time each week due to work or family commitments, here's how you can structure an efficient workout plan:

**Weekly Schedule Example:**

**Day 1 – Flexibility & Core Work (30 minutes)**

- o Dynamic warm-up
- o Planks (3 sets of 20–30 seconds)
- o Russian Twists (3 sets of 10 reps per side)
- o Static stretching

**Day 2 – Strength & Balance Training (45 minutes)**

- o Warm-up with dynamic stretches
- o Bodyweight squats/lunges
- o Single-leg balance drills
- o Dumbbell rows

**Day 3 – Cardiovascular Fitness & Recovery (30–60 minutes)**

- o Brisk walk around the neighborhood or light jogging
- o Foam rolling session targeting sore muscles

**Optional Rest Days:**

Allow at least one rest day per week where no strenuous activity occurs—this aids recovery.

## Tips for Staying Consistent

1. Start small: Commit to just two workouts per week initially if you're new to exercise.

2. Track progress: Keep notes on how long you hold planks or how many reps you complete—it's motivating!

The Journey Begins

3.  Make it fun: Choose activities you enjoy so that working out doesn't feel like a chore.

4.  Listen to your body: If something feels painful or uncomfortable beyond normal soreness levels after exercise sessions—stop immediately!

## Conclusion

By focusing on flexibility/mobility exercises alongside core strengthening routines balanced with cardiovascular conditioning—you'll be better prepared physically whether competing casually against friends or aiming towards personal best scores. Remember consistency matters more than intensity when starting out so stick with a plan outlined above while gradually increasing the difficulty overtime once you're comfortable with the basics already mastered.

# Understanding Golf's Unique Vocabulary

Golf, like many sports, has its own set of terms and phrases that can be confusing to those unfamiliar with the game. This specialized vocabulary serves not only to communicate effectively among players but also to create a sense of community and shared experience within the sport.

## The Importance of Golf Terminology

Knowing the language of golf is essential for anyone looking to engage fully with the game, whether as a player, parent, coach, or spectator. Terms such as "worm burner," "hosel rocket," and "coast to coast flight" are just a few examples of how golfers describe their shots, strategies, and experiences on the course. Understanding these terms allows players to discuss their games more intelligently and helps parents and spectators better appreciate the nuances of play.

## Building Connections Through Language

For many golfers, mastering this language is part of the social fabric of the sport. It fosters camaraderie among players who share similar experiences and challenges on the course. As one becomes more familiar with golf terminology, it opens up opportunities for deeper conversations about techniques, strategies, and even personal anecdotes related to golfing experiences.

In summary, understanding golf's unique vocabulary enhances both participation in and enjoyment of the game. It allows players to communicate effectively about their performance while also connecting with others who share their passion for golf.

## The Secret Language of Golf Revealed

**Above the Hole:** This term refers to the position of a golf ball on a sloping green. When a golfer's ball is located in such a way that the next putt will be downhill, it is described as being "above the hole." This positioning can significantly affect the difficulty of the subsequent putt, as downhill putts generally require more precision and control.

**Ace:** An "ace" is a term used in golf to denote a hole-in-one. This remarkable achievement occurs when a golfer successfully hits the ball directly from the tee into the hole on their very first stroke. Scoring an ace is considered one of the most exciting moments in golf and is celebrated among players.

**Address:** The term "address" refers to the final stance or position that a golfer assumes just before executing their swing at the ball. Proper addressing involves aligning oneself correctly with both the ball and the target, ensuring that grip, posture, and stance are all conducive to making an effective shot.

**Adjusted Gross Score:** The adjusted gross score (AGS) is your total score after factoring in your handicap stroke allowance. This adjustment helps create a level playing field among golfers of varying skill levels by allowing less skilled players additional strokes based on their handicap, thus making competitions fairer.

**Airmail:** In golfing slang, "airmail" describes a shot that travels well beyond its intended target area. For instance, if a player's approach shot overshoots the green and lands in rough terrain behind it, this would be referred to as having "airmailed" the green. Such shots can lead to challenging recovery situations for golfers.

**Albatross:** An albatross, commonly referred to as a double eagle, represents an extraordinary achievement in the sport of golf. It occurs when a golfer completes a par-5 hole in just two strokes, which is an exceptionally rare feat even among seasoned players.

**All Square:** This term is used in match play scoring to indicate that the match is tied. When both competitors have won an equal number of holes, the status of the match is described as "all square."

**Alternate Shot:** This format involves two players who take turns hitting the same golf ball until it is holed out. Each player alternates their shots throughout the round.

**Angle of Attack:** The angle of attack refers to the trajectory at which a golf club approaches the ball at impact. A steep angle of attack indicates a sharply downward motion, while a shallow angle suggests a flatter approach.

**Approach Shot:** A shot that is typically short to medium in distance, aimed at the putting green or the pin. This type of shot is commonly known as an "approach shot."

**Army Golf:** This term refers to a golfer whose shots frequently alternate between veering left and right, mimicking the movement pattern of soldiers marching (left, right, left).

**Attend the Flag:** A customary practice in golf where one player holds the flagstick in place and then removes it while another player prepares to putt.

**Attest:** In the context of tournament play, this term signifies the act of both a player and a fellow competitor signing a scorecard to verify that the recorded scores are correct.

**Away:** The phrase "You're away" indicates that a player's ball is the farthest from the hole, which typically means it is their turn to take a shot.

**Back Nine:** This term describes the final nine holes on an eighteen-hole golf course.

**Backspin:** This refers to the reverse spin that is applied to a golf ball, which helps prevent it from rolling forward after it lands on the green. This effect is often referred to as "bite," as it allows the ball to stop quickly upon landing.

**Back in the Stance:** This term describes a golfer's positioning of the ball closer to their back foot than their front foot during the address phase. This technique is commonly employed when hitting wedges, as it can help achieve a higher trajectory and better control over short shots.

**Bag Drop:** A bag drop is a designated area, typically located near the entrance of a clubhouse, where golfers can unload their clubs upon arrival. This allows players to leave their equipment while they find parking or prepare for their round.

**Ball Mark:** A ball mark is the indentation left on the green when a golf ball lands. It indicates where the ball has impacted the surface and can affect subsequent putts if not repaired properly.

**Ball Speed:** Ball speed is influenced by several factors, including the velocity of the club head at impact and how close to the sweet spot of the club face the ball was struck. Higher ball speeds generally result in greater distances traveled by the golf ball through the air.

**Ball Marker:** A ball marker is a small object used to indicate the position of a golf ball that has been lifted from the green. Common items such as coins are frequently utilized as ball markers.

**Banana Ball:** The term "banana ball" is a lighthearted slang expression referring to the trajectory of a golf ball that has been sliced. A slice occurs when the ball curves from left to right during its flight, resembling the shape of a banana.

**Barkie:** A "barkie" is a term used in golf to describe a situation where a golfer strikes a tree with their shot but still manages to achieve par on that hole.

**Beach [Bunker]:** In golfing terminology, "beach" or "bunker" refers to sand traps located on the course. These hazards are filled with sand, and players must be cautious not to ground their club before hitting the ball out of them.

**Bell:** A bell is utilized on golf fairways to signal when it is safe for groups behind to hit their approach shots, particularly after the group ahead has cleared the green. The ringing of the bell serves as an alert for players waiting to tee off or take their next shot.

**Below the Hole:** This term describes the location of a golf ball on a sloped green. When a golfer's ball is positioned such that the next putt will be uphill, it is referred to as being "below the hole." This positioning can influence putting strategy, as uphill putts generally require more force than downhill ones.

**Best Ball:** In this format, partners or teams play using only the best score recorded for each hole. Each golfer plays their own ball throughout the round, but at the end of each hole, only the lowest score among team members is counted as the team's score for that hole. This format encourages teamwork while allowing individual performance to shine.

**Birdie:** A birdie is achieved when a golfer scores one stroke under par on a specific hole. This indicates that the golfer performed exceptionally well relative to the expected standard for that hole.

**Bite:** The term "bite" refers to backspin applied to a golf ball, which causes it to stop quickly upon landing with minimal or no roll afterward. This technique is often used by golfers to control their shots and improve accuracy on approach shots and greens.

**Bladed Shot:** A bladed shot occurs when the club head makes improper contact with the ball, striking it at its equator with the leading edge of the club. This type of shot is also referred to as a "skulled" shot. As a result of this mishit, bladed shots tend to travel much lower and often farther than the golfer intended.

**Bogey:** In golf terminology, a bogey refers to a score that is one stroke over par for a specific hole. This indicates that the player took more strokes than the established par to complete that hole.

**Blind Draw:** A blind draw is a method used in competitions where players' names are randomly selected without prior knowledge or bias for pairing them together in matches.

**Break:** The term break describes the curvature or slope of a putting green, which influences how a putt will roll toward its target. This effect is caused by variations in elevation and the contours present on the green.

**Breakfast Ball:** The breakfast ball is an informal rule in golf that permits players to take an additional shot at their first tee-off without incurring any penalty. This practice is commonly accepted as a way to help golfers start their round on a positive note.

**Bunker:** A bunker is classified as a hazard on the golf course, typically characterized by a depression filled with sand. In some cases, bunkers may also be grassy depressions, serving as obstacles for players during their game.

**Buried Lie:** This term refers to a situation in golf where a ball is "plugged" or "embedded" either in a bunker or on any other part of the course. If the ball is embedded in the fairway or rough, the Rules of Golf permit the player to lift the ball and take relief without incurring a penalty. However, if the buried lie occurs within a penalty area or bunker, players are required to play the ball as it lies. Alternatively, they may declare it an "unplayable lie," which results in a one-stroke penalty.

**Cabbage:** This slang term describes extremely thick and deep rough that can be very difficult for golfers to escape from when their ball lands in it.

**Caddy:** A caddy is an individual who carries and manages a golfer's clubs during play. In addition to carrying equipment, caddies often assist players with selecting clubs and developing strategies for their shots.

**Car/Cart Fee:** This refers to the charge incurred for utilizing a golf cart during a round of golf.

**Car [or Golf Car]:** This term denotes the vehicle employed for transportation on a golf course. The two predominant types of golf cars are electric powered, which operate quietly, and gas-powered, which produce engine noise upon acceleration.

**Cart Path Only:** This is a temporary restriction that some golf clubs impose on golfers using carts. During inclement weather or wet conditions that could potentially harm the course, club management may require that cart drivers remain exclusively on designated paved cart paths throughout their round.

**Casting:** This term describes an early release of the wrist hinge during the downswing, resulting in a throwing motion that leads to a notable decrease in both power and control.

**Casual Water:** This term refers to any temporary accumulation of water on the golf course that is not classified as a water hazard and is visible either before or after a golfer takes their stance. If a player's ball lands in casual water, they are permitted to lift it and relocate it to the nearest point of relief without incurring any penalty.

**Chili-Dip:** A chili-dip occurs when a golfer mishits a chip shot by making contact with the ground before hitting the ball, resulting in a shot that travels only a short distance.

**Chicken Stick:** This term refers to a golfer's dependable club that they feel confident using to achieve solid contact and consistent performance on the course.

**CHIN:** An acronym for the Golf Handicap Information Network, CHIN is an online tool provided by the USGA that allows golfers to manage their handicaps by posting scores and maintaining an official handicap record.

**Chip Shot:** A chip shot is characterized as a short stroke with a low trajectory aimed at landing the ball on the green, allowing it to roll toward the hole upon landing.

**Chippie:** The term chippie describes the successful act of chipping the ball into the hole from around the green area.

**Chunk [Fat] Shots:** A chunk, often referred to as a "fat" shot, occurs when the golf club strikes the ground before making contact with the ball. This results in a significant divot being taken out of the turf, and typically leads to a shot that falls short of the intended target. The primary reason for this type of shot is usually improper swing mechanics or poor timing, where the player makes contact with the ground instead of hitting the ball cleanly.

**Thin [Skinny] Shots:** Conversely, a "thin" or "skinny" shot happens when the lower part of the clubface makes contact with the ball. This type of strike can propel the ball further than intended because it often results in less loft being applied to the shot. Players may experience thin shots due to an overly steep swing path or lifting their head too early during their swing.

**Clubhead Speed:** Clubhead speed refers to how quickly the club head is moving at the moment it strikes the golf ball, measured in miles per hour (mph). This metric is crucial because higher clubhead speeds generally lead to increased "ball speed," which significantly influences how far a golfer can hit the ball. Faster clubhead speeds allow for more energy transfer from the club to the ball, resulting in longer distances.

**Club Face:** The club face is located on the front part of the club head and features a flat surface that typically includes horizontal grooves designed to enhance grip on the ball upon impact. The angle and orientation of the club face at impact are vital for determining both direction and distance of each shot.

**Coast-to-Coast Flight:** This term refers to the act of hitting a golf ball from one bunker to another bunker across the green, demonstrating a notable lack of distance control.

**Compression:** When a fast-moving golf club strikes a golf ball, the ball undergoes a momentary compression, where it is partially "squished" by the clubface. This compression is not visible to the naked eye; however, high-speed photography has shown that the ball does indeed experience this phenomenon upon impact, which contributes to its subsequent flight at a high velocity.

**Condor:** A condor is defined as achieving a score of 4 under par on a single hole. This occurrence is exceedingly rare and can be likened to making a hole-in-one on a par-5 hole.

**Course Rating:** The Course Rating provides a numerical assessment of how challenging a golf course would be for a "scratch" golfer. It often differs from the total par of the course due to variations in overall length and difficulty level. For instance, if a golf course has a par of 72 but boasts a course rating of 73.2, it indicates that the course presents significant challenges, suggesting that an expert player would likely score above par.

**Clubhead:** The clubhead is the part of the golf club that is specifically designed for making contact with the golf ball. It is typically located at the end of the club and plays a crucial role in determining the direction, distance, and trajectory of the shot.

**Course:** In golf, the term "course" refers to the entire area designated for play. This encompasses all the holes, fairways, greens, roughs, hazards, and any other features that are part of a golf facility where players can engage in the game.

**Cut:** The term "cut" in golf has three distinct meanings:

1. **Shot Type:** The first meaning pertains to a specific type of shot characterized by a controlled movement from left to right. Unlike a slice—which is an unintended and often erratic shot—the cut is executed intentionally by golfers who aim for this particular trajectory.

2. **Grass Height Levels:** The second usage relates to the varying heights of grass on a golf course after a ball has exited the fairway. The "first cut" refers to the area of grass immediately adjacent to the fairway, which is slightly longer than that found on the fairway itself. In contrast, the "primary cut" denotes areas further away from the fairway where grass is significantly longer.

3. **Tournament Format:** The third definition involves tournament play, specifically referring to a 4-day event where players must achieve certain performance standards during initial rounds. Only those who meet or exceed these standards qualify to advance into subsequent rounds of competition.

**Daily Fee Course:** A high-quality public golf course that is owned privately but accessible to the general public without any restrictions.

**Dance Floor:** This term refers to the putting green, where golfers aim to position their balls as close to the hole as possible, representing the area where all the action in putting culminates.

**Defeated Flight:** This term describes a secondary group of players who have lost their matches in the first round of a tournament.

**Dew Sweeper:** A colloquial term for golfers who play early in the morning, often while there is still dew on the grass.

**Divots:** These are chunks of turf that are removed from the ground when a golfer strikes the ball. It is important for players to replace these divots and step on them, or if a seed mix is available (check your golf cart or tee box), to fill in the hole completely.

**Dogleg:** This term describes the configuration of golf holes that curve in one direction or another, resembling the bend in a dog's hind legs. When a hole curves to the right, it is designated as a "dogleg right," while a hole that curves to the left is known as a "dogleg left."

**Dormie:** In match play golf (as opposed to stroke play), a player or team is termed "dormie" when they are ahead by as many holes as there are holes left to play. For instance, if a player leads by three holes with three holes remaining, they are considered dormie.

**Double Bogey:** A double bogey indicates that a golfer has taken two strokes more than the par for that hole. For example, on a par-4 hole, scoring 6 would be classified as a double bogey. To minimize the risk of achieving this score, golfers should focus on avoiding penalty strokes.

**Double Cross:** This situation arises when a golfer plans to execute one type of shot (such as fading) but inadvertently hits another type (like hooking), resulting in unpredictable and often unfavorable outcomes.

**Double Eagle**: This term refers to a score that is three strokes under par on a specific hole. For instance, achieving a hole-in-one on a Par 4 hole qualifies as a double eagle, as does scoring 2 on a Par 5 hole. This remarkable achievement is also known as an Albatross and is recognized as the second rarest shot in golf, with estimated odds of occurring at approximately 6 million to 1.

**Down**: In the context of match play (a format where players compete to win individual holes), a player who has lost more holes than they have won is described as being "down" in the match. For example, if a player has won two holes but lost four, they are considered "two down." This terminology helps convey the current standing of players relative to each other during the match.

**Downswing**: The downswing represents the latter part of a full golf swing. After completing the backswing (the initial phase where the golfer raises the club), there is a transition where the golfer begins the downswing. This involves returning the club head towards the ball at high speed in preparation for impact, which is crucial for generating power and accuracy in the shot.

**Draw**: In golf, this term can refer to two concepts. Firstly, it describes a method of pairing players or teams for competitions (see "pairings"). Secondly, it denotes a specific ball flight pattern where the ball curves to the left (for right-handed golfers) during its trajectory.

**Drop**: A drop refers to the procedure of returning the ball to play after a player has taken relief from either a penalty area or an unplayable lie. To execute a drop, the player must hold the ball at knee height and allow it to fall freely to the ground. Once the ball has been dropped in this manner, it is deemed back in play.

**Driving Range**: Also known as the 'practice range,' this is a designated area on a golf course, or a separate facility specifically designed for golfers to practice their swings. Players can purchase bags or buckets of golf balls to hit, eliminating the need to retrieve them after each shot.

**Duck Hook**: A duck hook is an exaggerated version of a hook shot that results in the ball making a sharp turn to the left. This type of shot often elicits laughter from other players due to its extreme nature and unpredictability.

**Duff**: The term "duff" describes a poorly executed shot in golf, indicating that it was struck very badly (e.g., "He really duffed that shot."). The term has also led to the slang usage of "duffer," which refers to an unskilled golfer.

**Duffer**: A casual golfer who has not yet perfected their swing technique, resulting in higher scores during play. This type of golfer often enjoys the social aspect of the game, which may include consuming beer while on the course.

**Eagle**: An eagle is a golf score that occurs when a player completes a hole two strokes under par. Although still considered a rare accomplishment, eagles are more frequently achieved than holes-in-one (aces) or three-under-par scores (albatrosses). Typically, eagles are made on par-5 holes where a golfer can reach the green in two strokes and successfully make the putt.

**Elevated Green**: An elevated green refers to a putting surface that is situated higher than both the fairway and the surrounding terrain. Players must hit an uphill shot to reach this green, adding an extra challenge to their approach.

**Embedded Ball**: An embedded ball occurs when a golf ball lands in such a way that part of it sinks below ground level, becoming lodged in its own pitch mark. This situation can affect how players proceed with their next shot, as specific rules apply to embedded balls during play.

**Even Par:** This term refers to a scenario in golf where a player completes a hole using the same number of strokes as the hole's par rating, or when their total score for 18 holes equals the overall par rating for the entire course. For instance, if a golfer scores a 4 on a hole designated as a Par 4, this is classified as "even par." Similarly, achieving a total score of 72 on a course with a par of 72 is also considered even par.

**Executive Course:** An executive course is significantly shorter than a standard full-length 18-hole golf course. These courses typically feature shorter Par 3 and Par 4 holes, resulting in fewer total yards. This design allows players to complete their rounds in less time compared to traditional courses.

**Fade:** The fade, sometimes called a "cut," is characterized by a golf shot that exhibits a slight curve in its trajectory from left to right (for right-handed golfers). This type of shot can be strategically used to navigate around obstacles or position the ball favorably on the green.

**Fairway:** The fairway consists of closely mown grass that extends from the tee box to the green. It represents the ideal area for golfers to land their shots, as it provides optimal conditions for subsequent strokes.

**Fairway Woods:** Fairway woods are specialized golf clubs designed for longer shots. They are typically employed as the initial shot on shorter par 4 holes or for second shots on par 5 holes. While they resemble drivers, fairway woods have smaller club heads, are slightly shorter in length, and possess more loft, making them suitable for various situations on the course.

**Fat:** This term refers to a mishit golf shot where the club strikes the ground before making contact with the ball. This results in grass or dirt being interposed between the ball and the clubface, which significantly reduces the distance the ball travels. Such shots are often colloquially known as "chunked" shots.

**Flag Stick:** The flag stick is a movable pole that features a flag at its top, placed in the hole on the green. Its primary purpose is to indicate the location of the hole to players on the course.

**Flights:** In golf, flights refer to groups of players who are bracketed together based on their qualifying scores or seeding. This organization helps manage competitions by ensuring that players of similar skill levels compete against one another.

**Flop Shot:** A flop shot is characterized as a high and soft shot that lands gently on the green. Typically executed using a lob wedge or sand wedge, this type of shot requires considerable skill and precision, often associated with accomplished golfers such as Phil Mickelson.

**Flyer:** When grass gets between the club face and the ball, particularly on shots taken from the rough, it can reduce friction, which in turn diminishes the backspin applied to the ball. As a result, these shots may come out with increased velocity, travel farther than anticipated, and roll significantly after landing. This phenomenon is referred to as a "flyer."

**Fly The Green:** The phrase "fly the green" describes a golf shot that overshoots its intended target area entirely. For instance, if a golfer's approach shot lands well past the putting surface and into the rough behind it, this is termed as having "flown the green."

**Foot Wedge:** This humorous slang refers to an instance where a golfer uses their foot to nudge their ball from a challenging lie to make their next shot more manageable. It is widely recognized among golfers that this practice is against the rules of golf.

**Fore:** This term is shouted as a warning to alert others on the course that a player's ball is heading in their direction and could potentially hit someone.

**Forward Tees:** Most golf courses feature multiple tee boxes from which players can drive the ball. The "forward tees" are positioned closest to the fairway, resulting in the shortest overall length of the hole when players opt to tee off from these boxes.

**Four Jack:** This term is slang for a situation in which a golfer takes four putts to complete a hole, indicating a struggle with putting.

**Foursome:** This term refers to a group of four golfers playing together during a round of golf. In contrast, a "threesome" denotes three golfers, a "twosome" indicates two golfers, and "single" refers to one golfer playing alone.

**Free Drop:** Under specific circumstances outlined in the Rules of Golf, players are allowed to relocate their ball without incurring a penalty stroke. The Rules also specify how this "free drop" should be executed.

**Fried Egg:** A "fried egg" in golf refers to a challenging situation where the ball is partially buried in a bunker, resembling the appearance of a fried egg. This scenario demands a high level of skill and finesse from the golfer, as executing a successful shot can be difficult due to the need to generate spin while dealing with the sand's resistance.

**Fringe:** The fringe is an area of grass that surrounds the green, typically cut slightly higher than the grass on the green itself. While landing on the fringe does not count as being on the green in regulation play, golfers often treat it similarly when putting. A common technique used on or around the fringe is the chip shot, where players utilize a wedge to gently bump and roll the ball towards the hole.

**Frog Hair:** Commonly referred to as "fringe," frog hair describes the strip of grass that encircles the putting surface. The height of frog hair is longer than that of the grass on the green but shorter than that found in the rough areas adjacent to it. This distinction helps golfers understand how to approach shots taken from this area.

**Front Nine:** The term "Front Nine" denotes the first nine holes of an 18-hole golf course. Specifically, holes numbered 1 through 9 are categorized as the Front Nine, while holes numbered 10 through 18 are known as the Back Nine. Understanding this division is essential for golfers when discussing their rounds or strategizing their play.

**Gimme:** A "gimme" in golf refers to a short putt that players agree can be counted as made without the need for the player to actually hit the ball into the hole. This informal agreement is typically based on the proximity of the ball to the hole, and it serves as a courtesy among players, allowing them to save time and effort during a round.

**Golf:** The term "golf" has its origins in Scotland, where it first appeared in a statute from 1457. The word is believed to derive from an older concept meaning "to strike" or "to cuff." Golf is played on a specially designed course and involves hitting a ball into a series of holes using clubs, with the objective being to complete each hole in as few strokes as possible.

**Golf Bag:** A golf bag is an essential accessory for golfers, typically made from materials such as leather, vinyl, or canvas. It is designed to carry golf clubs, balls, and various accessories needed during play. Golf bags come in different styles, including stand bags and cart bags, catering to different preferences and playing conditions.

**Golf Glove:** A golf glove is worn primarily on the left hand (for right-handed players) to enhance grip on the club. Wearing a glove helps prevent slippage during swings, especially in adverse weather conditions like rain or when hands are sweaty. This added grip contributes significantly to better control and accuracy while playing.

**Golf Shoes:** Golf shoes are specifically engineered footwear designed for playing golf. They feature specialized soles that provide traction necessary for maintaining balance during swings while also ensuring comfort throughout the game. The design of golf shoes often includes spikes or other gripping mechanisms that help prevent slipping on grass surfaces.

**Grand Slam**: The PGA Tour's four major championships consist of the Masters, the U.S. Open, the PGA Championship, and The Open Championship. A player who wins all four of these prestigious events within a single calendar year is recognized as having achieved the "Grand Slam."

**Green**: This area of the golf hole is specifically designed for putting and represents the most meticulously maintained section of the golf course.

**Greens Fee**: This term refers to the fixed amount that a golf club charges players for access to its course, allowing them to play either 9 or 18 holes.

**Green In Regulation (GIR)**: Commonly abbreviated as GIR, this statistic indicates when a golfer reaches the green in the expected number of strokes relative to par. For example, a player achieves GIR by reaching the green in one stroke on a Par 3 hole, in two strokes on a Par 4 hole, or in three strokes on a Par 5 hole.

**Greenskeeper**: This individual is responsible for maintaining and caring for the golf course. Their duties include mowing grass, managing irrigation systems, applying fertilizers and pesticides, and ensuring overall course quality.

**Grip**: The grip refers to the portion of the golf club that a golfer holds. Common materials used for grips include leather and rubber, which provide varying levels of comfort and traction. Additionally, the term "grip" encompasses how a golfer positions their hands on the club, which is crucial for effective swing mechanics.

**Grooves**: Grooves are the horizontal indentations found on the face of a golf club. Their primary function is to enhance friction when the club strikes the ball, enabling the ball to achieve backspin during its flight. This backspin can significantly affect the ball's trajectory and landing behavior on the green.

**Grounding Your Club**: Grounding your club involves allowing the club head to make contact with the ground behind the ball before initiating your swing. According to golf rules, players are permitted to ground their clubs in areas such as fairways or roughs; however, this practice is not allowed when the ball is situated in a sand trap.

**Ground Under Repair**: This term refers to any section of a golf course that has been designated by course management as unplayable. Such areas are typically marked with white paint, indicating that players must remove their balls from these zones and drop them at the nearest point of relief without incurring any penalties.

**Gross Score:** A player's gross score refers to the total number of strokes taken during their round of golf, without any modifications for handicap calculations.

**Hacker:** This term is used pejoratively to describe a golfer who possesses limited skills and typically has a high handicap, indicating their level of play. Hackers may also be called "duffers."

**Handicap:** A golf handicap is a numerical measure that reflects a player's average performance relative to par, allowing golfers of varying abilities to compete on an equitable basis.

**Hazard:** In golf terminology, a "hazard" encompasses any area such as bunkers or water hazards that poses a challenge to players.

**Head-to-Head**: This term refers to the competition between two players or teams, evaluated on a hole-by-hole basis. It is commonly known as match play, where each hole is treated as a separate contest, and the player or team that wins the most holes wins the match.

**Heel**: In golf terminology, the heel is the part of the club face that is located closest to where the golf shaft connects to the club head. This area is crucial for understanding how different strikes can affect ball trajectory and distance. The opposite end of the club face is known as the "toe."

**Hit**: The term "hit" describes when a player makes contact with the golf ball. It encompasses various types of strokes, particularly distinguishing between a controlled stroke, such as putting, and a more aggressive hit that may lack precision and distance control. The latter often occurs when a player rushes their putt.

**Hole**: A hole in golf consists of several components: it includes a teeing ground from which players start their play, a putting green where the hole is located, and all areas in between. Additionally, "hole" can refer specifically to the physical hole on the green into which players aim to sink their ball.

**Hole-In-One**: A hole-in-one occurs when a golfer successfully hits their tee shot directly into the hole with just one stroke. This remarkable achievement is also referred to as an ace and is celebrated for its rarity and skill involved.

**Honor:** The term "honor" refers to the player who is designated to tee off first on a hole in golf. This is typically determined by the order of play established at the start of the round or based on the score from the previous hole.

**Hook:** A hook is a type of shot that curves the ball from right to left in the air, primarily affecting right-handed golfers. This occurs when the clubface is closed relative to the swing path at impact, causing the ball to spin in a way that results in this leftward trajectory. While a hook can generate additional distance due to topspin, it can also lead to undesirable outcomes, such as a severe misdirection known as a duck-hook. A less pronounced version of a hook is referred to as a draw or push-draw, which still curves left but with less severity.

**Hosel:** The hosel is an integral part of a golf club, specifically located at the top of the club head where the shaft is inserted. It serves as a connection point between the shaft and club head and can be described as an open hole or socket-like structure. In some designs, particularly those where the hosel and clubhead are manufactured as one piece, it may refer more broadly to this area.

**Hosel Rocket:** The term "hosel rocket" is slang for what is known as a shank in golfing terminology. A shank occurs when a player mishits the ball by striking it off the hosel of the club head rather than its face.

This results in an erratic shot that travels very low and veers sharply to the right (for right-handed players), often leading to frustration for golfers.

**Hybrid:** A hybrid golf club combines features from both fairway woods and long irons, making it easier for players to hit than traditional long irons. Hybrids are designed with characteristics that enhance forgiveness and playability, allowing golfers to achieve better distance and accuracy from various lies on the course.

**Impact Position:** This refers to the alignment and posture of your body at the precise moment when your club strikes the ball. For optimal ball striking, various parts of your body—such as your hands, wrists, elbows, arms, shoulders, hips, and both upper and lower body—should be positioned according to established guidelines at the moment of impact.

**In Play:** After a golfer takes a shot from the tee box, the ball is considered "in play." It remains in this status until it is either successfully holed out, lost, marked, and lifted (when on the putting green), or struck out of bounds.

**Interlocking Grip:** This term describes a specific technique for gripping the golf club. In this method, the golfer interlaces their hands by placing the index finger of their lead hand between the pinky and ring fingers of their trailing hand. This creates an "interlocked" grip that can enhance control and stability during swings.

**In the Leather**: This term refers to a situation in golf where a short putt is considered so close to the hole that it can be conceded as made without actually being putted. Specifically, if the distance remaining for the putt is less than approximately 24 inches (the distance from the putter head to the bottom of the grip), it is said to be "in the leather." This concession is typically only applicable during friendly or unofficial rounds of golf.

**Iron**: The term "irons" encompasses all golf clubs with heads usually made of steel, designed for shots that are generally 200 yards or less, particularly for amateur players. Irons are distinct from woods, which are used primarily for longer shots such as drives.

**Kick-In**: A kick-in refers to an extremely short putt, often less than one foot from the hole, which is virtually impossible to miss. Due to its proximity, golfers typically consider these putts automatic.

**Knee Knocker**: This phrase describes a short putt that a golfer would normally expect to make but may feel anxious about due to pressure or nerves in critical moments. The psychological aspect of putting can turn what should be a straightforward shot into a challenging one.

**Knickers**: Often known as "Plus Fours," knickers are loose-fitting golf trousers that are cut short and gathered at the knee. These garments were particularly fashionable in the early 19th and 20th centuries but have largely fallen out of favor on modern golf courses.

**Lag Putt**: A lag putt refers to a long putt where the golfer does not realistically expect to make the shot. Instead, the objective is to get the ball as close to the hole as possible, minimizing the distance for the next putt.

**Lateral Hazard**: A lateral hazard is defined as a water hazard, such as a stream or pond, that runs alongside or parallel to the line of play towards the hole. These hazards are typically marked with red stakes on the golf course.

**Launch Angle**: The launch angle describes the angle at which a golf ball ascends vertically immediately after being struck by a club. This angle is measured in degrees relative to the ground and plays a crucial role in determining how high and far the ball will travel.

**Lay Up:** This is a strategic golf shot where the player intentionally strikes the ball a shorter distance than what might typically be expected. The purpose of this tactic is to steer clear of hazards or challenging areas on the course, thereby simplifying the next shot.

**Lead Foot or Hand:** This term describes the part of the golfer's body—be it foot, hand, or another area—that is closest to the target during the setup phase when preparing to hit the ball.

**Level Par:** This phrase indicates a score that matches the course's par. For instance, if a golfer completes a round with a score of 72 and the course par is also 72, that golfer is said to have achieved level par.

**Line:** In golf, this term refers to the theoretical trajectory on the putting green that extends from the golfer's ball to the hole, outlining how the putt will travel.

**Lie:** In golf, the term "lie" has two primary meanings. The first refers to the position of the golf ball in relation to the ground. For example, a ball that is sitting in thick grass or deep rough can be described as having a "thick lie," while a ball that is partially buried in the ground may be referred to as a "plugged lie." The second meaning pertains to the angle of the club shaft compared to the sole of the club, which affects how the club interacts with the ground during a swing.

**Links:** This term can denote flat European-style golf courses characterized by expansive greens. Additionally, it can simply refer to the act of playing a round of golf, regardless of course type.

**Lip Out:** A "lip out" occurs when a putt seems destined for success but veers off course at the last moment, failing to enter the hole. A less frustrating variant of this situation is known as a "burnt edge," where the ball grazes the edge of the hole but does not drop in.

**Loft:** The term "loft" describes the angle formed between the face of a golf club and the ground. Clubs with higher loft angles will launch the ball higher into the air upon impact, making loft an important factor in determining how far and high a shot will travel.

**Long Game**: The "long game" in golf refers to the category of shots that are executed from a distance greater than 100 yards from the green. This aspect of the game emphasizes power and accuracy, as players must navigate longer distances while considering factors such as wind, elevation changes, and course layout. In contrast, the "short game" encompasses all shots taken from within 100 yards of the green, focusing on precision and finesse.

**Lost Ball**: A lost ball is defined as one that a golfer cannot locate after it has been struck. According to the Rules of Golf, players are permitted to search for a lost ball for a maximum of three minutes. If the ball remains unfound after this period, specific procedures must be followed, including taking a penalty stroke and dropping a new ball in accordance with established rules.

**LPGA: Teaching & Club Professional [T&CP] Division**: This division represents a crucial segment of the Ladies Professional Golf Association (LPGA), which is recognized as one of the leading women's sports organizations globally. The T&CP Division focuses on promoting golf education and professional development for women in teaching and club management roles.

**LPGA: Ladies Professional Golf Association**: The LPGA is noted for being the longest-running women's sports association in history, having celebrated its 50th anniversary in 2000. It plays a vital role in advancing women's participation in golf at all levels, from amateur to professional competitions.

**Match Play**: Match play is a competitive format where individual players compete directly against one another rather than against an entire field. In this format, players earn points based on their performance on each hole; specifically, they receive one point for each hole won against their opponent.

**Medal Play:** Also known as "stroke play," medal play is a golf scoring format where the player totals all the strokes taken during their round. The final score is simply the cumulative number of strokes recorded.

**Medalist:** This term refers to the player who achieves the lowest gross score during qualifying rounds.

**Mixed Foursome:** This format involves teams that include both male and female golfers, typically consisting of two men and two women.

**Mulligan:** A mulligan allows golfers to retake a shot if they are dissatisfied with the initial outcome. While this practice is often accepted in casual games among friends, it is not permitted in official tournaments, where taking a mulligan would incur a penalty.

**Nassau**: This term refers to a specific type of wager in golf that combines three distinct bets into one. In a Nassau bet, participants place money on three outcomes: the best score on the front nine holes, the best score on the back nine holes, and the overall best score for the entire 18-hole round.

**Net Score**: A player's net score is calculated by totaling all strokes taken during a round or on individual holes and then subtracting the player's handicap from this total. The handicap is a numerical measure of a golfer's potential ability, allowing players of varying skill levels to compete fairly against one another.

**Nineteenth Hole**: This colloquial term refers to the bar or restaurant where golfers often gather after completing their round. It serves as a social hub for players to relax, discuss their game, and enjoy refreshments.

**Open Face**: In golfing terminology, an "open face" occurs when the club head is angled to the right of the target line at impact. Additionally, it can describe a club head that is positioned significantly upward when preparing to execute a high lob shot.

**Open Stance**: An open stance describes a golfer's alignment at address where their feet and body are positioned so that they are aimed left of their intended target line. This stance can affect swing mechanics and shot trajectory.

**Out of Bounds:** Golf courses typically feature markers such as ground stakes and fences that delineate the boundaries of the course. If a player's ball lands outside these designated indicators, it is considered "out of bounds."

**Overlapping Grip:** The overlapping grip is a technique for holding the golf club where the pinky finger of the lower hand rests in the groove between the index and middle fingers of the upper hand. This grip is sometimes known as the "Vardon grip," named after the famous golfer Harry Vardon.

**Pace of Play:** Pace of play refers to how quickly a group completes their round of golf. A common guideline is to maintain a speed that keeps you in line with the group ahead.

**Pairing Sheet:** A pairing sheet is a document that lists the pairings, or groups, of players participating in a tournament round of golf.

**Pairings:** Pairings refer to the individuals with whom players are grouped during a tournament round of golf.

**Par:** A golfer achieves a par on a hole when the number of strokes taken equals the par value assigned to that hole. For instance, if a golfer scores 4 on a hole designated as Par 4, this is considered a par score. Similarly, scoring 5 on a Par 5 hole also qualifies as a par.

**Penalty Stroke:** A penalty stroke is an additional stroke added to a player's score due to a violation of the rules. The specific situations that warrant these penalty strokes are outlined in the Rules of Golf, which detail various infractions and their corresponding penalties.

**Pin:** Commonly referred to as the "flag stick," the pin is a metal pole topped with a colored flag that marks the location of the hole on the green. This helps golfers gauge their distance from the hole during play.

**Pin High:** The term "pin high" describes an approach shot that lands at the same depth on the green as the flag stick. This indicates that the golfer has accurately judged the distance for their shot, landing it near where they intended.

**Pitch Shot:** A pitch shot is characterized as a short game shot typically played from approximately 40 to 60 yards away from the hole. It is executed with a high trajectory, allowing for minimal roll upon landing on the green due to its steep descent.

**Pitch Mark:** A pitch mark is an indentation created on the putting green when a golf ball lands. It is considered proper golf etiquette for players to repair any pitch marks they create to maintain the quality of the green.

**PGA of America:** Established in 1916, the PGA of America is the largest sports organization globally, with over 28,000 members dedicated to promoting golf across various demographics and regions.

**PGA Tour:** The PGA Tour refers to the professional golf tour that features many of the top golfers in the world, which is commonly broadcasted on television.

**Pitch Shot:** A pitch shot is a short golf shot characterized by a high trajectory that allows the ball to land softly on the green with minimal roll afterward.

**Play Through:** When golfers recognize that their pace of play is slower than expected and are holding up the group behind them, it is courteous for them to allow that group to "play through" by stepping aside and letting them proceed ahead.

**Plugged Lie:** This term describes a situation in golf where a ball becomes partially embedded in the ground after landing in its own pitch mark. According to the Rules of Golf, players are permitted to take relief without penalty from a plugged lie, with the exception of sand traps.

**Plus Golfer:** This term refers to an exceptionally skilled golfer whose handicap is less than zero. Unlike less skilled golfers who subtract their handicap strokes from their total score, a plus golfer must add strokes to their total score when participating in net events.

**Practice Putting Green:** This is a designated area on a golf course specifically set aside for players to practice their putting skills.

**Preferred Lie:** This term is used when course conditions are not optimal, prompting the manager or head professional to implement a local rule that allows players to improve their lie. This typically involves the "lift, clean, and place" rule, which permits players to lift their ball, clean it, and place it back in a more favorable position before making their shot.

**Private Golf Course:** A private golf course is one where access is limited strictly to members and their guests only, restricting play from the general public.

**Provisional Ball:** If you suspect that your ball may be lost or out of bounds after playing a shot, it is advisable to play a second ball immediately as a provisional. This approach is efficient because if you later find out that your original ball is indeed lost, you will not need to return to the original spot to hit again, thus saving time on the course.

**Public Golf Course:** A public golf course is one that allows members of the general public to play by paying a greens fee or daily fee. These courses are accessible to anyone who wishes to play golf, without the need for membership in a private club.

**Push/Pull:** Pushes and pulls refer to inaccurate golf shots that do not travel along the intended target line. For right-handed golfers, a push occurs when the ball travels to the right of the aimed target, while a pull occurs when it goes to the left. Typically, both types of shots result in straight ball flight rather than the curved trajectories associated with slices or hooks.

**Punch Shot:** A punch shot is characterized by a significantly lower trajectory than usual for a golf shot. This type of shot is often executed intentionally by players aiming to keep the ball beneath wind conditions or tree branches.

**Putt**: A putt is a specific type of golf shot executed when the ball is on the green. The player uses a specialized golf club known as a putter to strike the ball, aiming to make it roll smoothly along the ground toward the hole. The objective is to either sink the ball directly into the cup or position it very close to it for an easier subsequent shot.

**Putter**: The putter is the designated golf club utilized for making putts, particularly when the ball is on or in close proximity to the putting surface. This club is designed with a flat face and a heavier head compared to other clubs, allowing for precise control and accuracy needed for short-distance shots.

**Quad Bogey**: A quad bogey denotes a score that exceeds par by four strokes on any given hole. For instance, if a golfer scores 8 on a Par 4 hole, this would be classified as a quad bogey. Similarly, scoring 9 on a Par 5 hole would also result in a quad bogey.

**Range**: The term "range," abbreviated from "driving range," refers to an area designated for golfers to practice their swings. Driving ranges are typically located adjacent to golf courses and may be part of a larger golf club facility; however, they can also exist as independent commercial venues where golfers pay per bucket of balls to practice their skills.

**Range Finder**: A range finder is an electronic device designed to assist golfers in measuring the distance from their current position to a specific target on the golf course. These devices utilize laser technology, where a laser beam is directed towards the target. Upon reaching the target, the beam reflects back to the range finder, allowing it to calculate and display the precise yardage to that point.

This technology enhances a golfer's ability to make informed decisions regarding club selection and shot strategy based on accurate distance measurements.

**Reading The Green**: Each putting green features various undulations and slopes, which can subtly influence the path of a golf ball as it rolls toward the hole. The process of analyzing these contours to predict how they will affect an upcoming putt is known as "reading the green." Golfers carefully observe factors such as slope direction, grain of the grass, and any imperfections on the surface that could alter the ball's trajectory. Mastering this skill is crucial for improving putting accuracy and overall performance on the green.

**Ready Golf**: To promote an efficient Pace of Play during rounds of golf, players within a group are encouraged to adopt a "ready golf" approach. This means that golfers should play their shots when they are prepared to do so, rather than adhering strictly to traditional order based on who is farthest from the hole. By allowing players to hit when ready, this practice can help reduce delays and keep the game moving smoothly.

**Relief**: In certain circumstances outlined by the Rules of Golf, players are permitted to move their ball without incurring a penalty. One common scenario is when a ball lies in an area designated as "ground under repair." When golfers reposition their ball according to these rules—such as moving it out of an unplayable lie or taking relief from obstructions—they are said to be "taking relief." Understanding when and how relief can be taken is essential for maintaining fair play and adhering to golfing regulations.

**Re-load:** This term is used in golf slang to describe the action of a player taking a second shot immediately after hitting a poor first shot.

The Journey Begins

It is commonly referenced on the tee box, particularly when a golfer's initial tee shot goes out of bounds.

**Resort:** A golf course that is situated in a vacation or destination area, often associated with accommodations for visitors. These courses typically cater to tourists and may offer various amenities alongside golfing.

**Reverse Pivot:** In an ideal golf swing for right-handed players, weight is shifted to the right during the backswing and then transferred back to the left during the downswing. A "reverse pivot" occurs when this weight shift is performed incorrectly, meaning the player shifts their weight left on the backswing and right on the downswing.

**Rough:** This refers to areas of longer grass that border the fairways and extend from the tee box to the green. Golfers generally aim to avoid landing their ball in the rough due to its challenging playing conditions.

**Round:** The standard format of playing golf consists of eighteen holes.

**Rub of the Green:** The official definition of "rub of the green" refers to "the accidental deflection of a ball in motion by an outside agency." Over time, this term has evolved to encompass a broader interpretation, often used to signify any instance of bad luck experienced by a golfer during play.

**Sand Trap:** A sand trap is defined as a man-made depression filled with sand, strategically placed along fairways or near greens. These features are designed to increase the difficulty of play, compelling golfers to navigate around them. Players typically aim to avoid these hazards, which are also commonly known as "bunkers."

**Sandbagger:** This term is used derogatorily to describe a golfer who intentionally misrepresents their skill level by inflating their handicap. The purpose of this deception is to gain an unfair advantage in betting situations during competitive events.

**Sand Save:** This term describes the scenario where a golfer successfully makes par after hitting from a greenside bunker. Achieving this feat is often referred to colloquially as making a "sandy," highlighting the skill required to recover from such challenging positions on the course.

**Sandy**: A "sandy" refers to a situation in golf where a player successfully makes par after hitting their ball out of a greenside bunker. This achievement is often called a "sand save."

**Scramble Format**: In this format, each member of a team takes a tee shot. The team then selects the best shot among them and plays the next stroke from that location. This process continues, with the team repeatedly choosing the best shot until they hole out. The score for each hole is recorded, and the cumulative score is tallied as the team's overall score.

**Seeding**: Seeding involves arranging players in a draw based on their skill levels to ensure fair competition.

**Scratch**: A scratch golfer is an exceptionally skilled player whose handicap is 0, meaning they do not require any additional strokes to match the Course Rating on any golf course.

**Skulled Shot**: This term is synonymous with "bladed shot," which refers to a type of mishit where the ball is struck too high on the clubface, resulting in low trajectory and excessive distance.

186

**Semi-Private Golf Course**: A semi-private golf course has both members who pay for exclusive access and allows limited public play, providing a mix of private and public golfing experiences.

**Shaft:** The shaft of a golf club is the elongated, tapered tube that connects the grip to the club head. In general, shafts for drivers and fairway woods are predominantly constructed from graphite due to its lightweight and flexible properties, which can enhance swing speed and distance. Conversely, iron shafts are typically made from steel, providing greater durability and control.

**Shank:** The shank, often referred to as "The S Word" among golfers, is a particularly dreaded mishit. It occurs when the ball is struck off the neck or heel of the club, resulting in a shot that veers sharply to the right (for right-handed golfers). Shanks can be psychologically challenging for players because they are often perceived as contagious; many golfers believe that simply mentioning them can lead to an increased likelihood of experiencing one.

**Short Game:** The short game encompasses all types of shots executed within 100 yards of the green. This includes various techniques such as pitches (high shots with a soft landing), chips (low shots that roll out), bunker shots (played from sand traps), and putts (striking the ball on the green towards the hole). Mastery of the short game is crucial for lowering scores, as it involves precision and touch.

**Short-Sided:** The term "short-sided" describes a situation where a golfer hits an approach shot to the same side of the green where the pin is located. This positioning complicates subsequent chips or pitches because there is less green to work with for landing the ball softly before it rolls toward the hole.

**Shot:** In golf terminology, a shot refers to the action of striking a golf ball with a club. Each individual strike is considered either a shot or stroke, contributing to a player's overall score during a round.

**Shotgun Start**: A shotgun start is a golf tournament format where all groups of players begin their rounds simultaneously from different holes on the course. This method allows for a more efficient use of time, as it enables all participants to complete their rounds in a similar timeframe rather than waiting for each group to tee off sequentially from the first hole.

**Skinny**: The term "skinny" in golf refers to a mishit shot that occurs when the very bottom edge of the club face makes contact with the ball. This type of shot is also known as hitting the ball "thin." It typically happens when the golfer's club head moves upward through impact instead of descending at the correct angle. As a result, these shots often lead to lower trajectory and less distance than intended.

**Skins**: In a skins game, golfers compete within their foursome by aiming to achieve the lowest score on each hole. The player who has the lowest score on a hole wins that hole's "skin," which is usually associated with a predetermined monetary value (for example, $1 or $5). If multiple players tie for the lowest score on a hole, that skin carries over to the next hole, increasing its value.

**Slice**: A slice is a common problem faced by amateur golfers, characterized by a shot that curves dramatically from left to right in mid-air. This phenomenon occurs due to excessive sidespin imparted on the ball during impact, resulting in reduced distance and accuracy. A less severe version of this issue may be referred to as a cut or pull-cut.

The Journey Begins

**Slope Rating**: The slope rating quantifies the difficulty of a golf course specifically for amateur players, with values ranging from 55 to 155. A higher slope rating indicates a more challenging course.

**Snowman**: The term "snowman" is used in golf to describe a score of 8 on a player's scorecard. This term is derived from the visual appearance of the number 8, which resembles a snowman. Scoring a snowman can significantly affect a player's overall performance in a round.

**Sole**: The sole refers to the bottom part of a golf club's head that makes contact with the ground when the club is at address. It runs from the toe (the front part) to the heel (the back part) and includes both the leading edge (the front edge) and trailing edge (the back edge).

**Slope**: Slope is a numerical value that indicates how difficult a golf course is for a bogey golfer compared to a scratch golfer. This rating plays an essential role in calculating a golfer's handicap index, helping to level the playing field among golfers of varying skill levels.

**Stableford**: This is a scoring system used in golf where points are awarded based on the number of strokes taken on each hole, rather than simply counting total strokes. For example, a bogey (one stroke over par) earns 1 point, while a par (equal to par) earns 2 points, and a birdie (one stroke under par) earns 3 points. This system encourages players to play aggressively and can lead to more enjoyable rounds since it allows for better scoring opportunities even if a player has a bad hole.

**Stance**: The stance in golf refers to how a golfer positions their feet relative to each other when addressing the ball. It is typically categorized as square (feet parallel to the target line), open (front foot further from the target), or closed (back foot further from the target). Additionally, the stance can be described by how wide or narrow it is, which can affect balance and swing mechanics.

**Sticks**: In golfing slang, "sticks" refers to golf clubs. This informal term is commonly used among golfers when discussing their equipment or during casual conversations about the game.

**Stimpmeter**: The stimpmeter is an instrument designed to measure the speed of putting greens. It resembles a yardstick with a V-shaped groove along its length. To use it, one end of the stimpmeter is elevated while a golf ball is rolled down its track onto the green. The distance that the ball travels on the putting surface determines the Stimp Rating for that green, providing valuable information about its speed for players and course managers alike.

**Stinger**: A stinger is a specific type of golf shot characterized by a very low trajectory. This shot is typically executed from the tee box and is particularly useful in situations where there is a headwind or when the ground conditions are firm, allowing the ball to roll significantly after landing.

**Stroke**: In golf, the term "stroke" refers to the action of striking the golf ball with a club. It can also be referred to as a shot.

**Stroke Play**: Stroke play is a format of golf where the total score for a completed stipulated round is counted. This format is commonly known as "medal play."

**Strong Grip**: A strong grip in golf involves positioning the hands on the club such that the 'V' shapes formed between the thumbs and forefingers point towards the golfer's right shoulder. Additionally, this grip allows the golfer to see more than two knuckles of their left hand at address.

The Journey Begins

**Superintendent**: The superintendent is responsible for maintaining the golf course, ensuring its overall health and playability. This individual may also be referred to as the greenskeeper.

**Sweet Spot:** The sweet spot refers to a specific area on the club face of a golf club that optimally transfers energy to the golf ball upon impact. When the ball strikes this precise location, it results in minimal vibration felt in the club, leading to a more effective and powerful shot.

**Swing:** In golf, the full swing encompasses a series of intricate and coordinated movements executed by the golfer to strike the ball. This sequence includes four main components: the backswing (the initial movement away from the ball), the downswing (the motion bringing the club down towards the ball), the follow-through (the continuation of movement after hitting the ball), and finally, the finish (the position at which the swing concludes).

**Swing Path:** This term describes the trajectory or direction in which the club head travels as it approaches and makes contact with the golf ball. Swing paths can be categorized into three primary types: "outside-in" (where the club moves from outside to inside relative to the target line), "inside-out" (where it moves from inside to outside), and "down the line" (where it travels straight along the intended target line).

**Swing Plane:** The swing plane is an imaginary flat surface that represents the angle formed during both backswing and follow-through. It serves as a guide for maintaining proper swing mechanics, helping golfers achieve consistency in their shots.

**Takeaway:** The takeaway is the initial phase of the backswing in golf, beginning when the club head is positioned behind the ball at address.

This phase continues until the club reaches a point where it is parallel to the ground and aligned with the target path, a position referred to as double parallel.

**Tap In:** A tap-in is a very short putt that is considered nearly impossible to miss. It is often colloquially known as a gimme or a kick-in, indicating that it requires minimal effort to complete.

**Tee:** A tee is a small device made of wood or plastic that elevates the golf ball off the ground. Tees are primarily used when playing from the tee box at the start of each hole.

**Tee Box [or teeing ground]:** The tee box is a specific area on each golf course hole designated for players to take their first shot. Most courses feature multiple tee boxes per hole, allowing golfers of varying skill levels to select the most suitable option for their game.

**Tee Shot:** A tee shot refers to the first stroke taken from the tee box on every hole, marking the beginning of play for that particular hole.

**Tee Time:** This refers to the scheduled time for starting a round of golf. For instance, if you have a tee time at nine o'clock, it indicates that you should be ready to tee off on the first hole at exactly 9:00 AM.

**Tempo:** This term describes the rhythm and pace of a golfer's swing, which can be somewhat subjective. It is often characterized by descriptors such as fast, slow, or smooth. Each golfer has a unique tempo that reflects their individual style and approach to swinging the club.

**Tending The Flag:** Historically in golf, it was required to remove the flagstick from the hole before a putt could be made. This process involved a playing partner holding the flagstick while another player putted and then removing it as the ball approached the hole. This action was known as "tending the flag."

**Texas Wedge:** This is a colloquial term used when a golfer chooses to use their putter for a shot taken from off the green instead of using a wedge for chipping. It typically occurs when the ball is close enough to the green that putting is deemed more effective than chipping.

**Thin:** The optimal golf shot occurs when the club face makes contact with the bottom part of the ball, which is resting on the ground. However, due to various swing imperfections, golfers may strike the ball higher up, near its equator. This type of mishit is commonly referred to as hitting the ball "thin."

**The Tips:** Golf courses typically feature multiple tee boxes. The forward tees are designed to provide an easier and shorter route to the hole, while the back tees, known as "the tips," present a more challenging and longer path. It is generally recommended that only the most skilled players attempt to play from these back tees.

**The Turn:** An 18-hole golf course is divided into two sections: the front nine (the first nine holes) and the back nine (the last nine holes). When a player finishes playing the front nine and prepares to start on the back nine, this transition is referred to as "making the turn."

**Tight Lie:** A "tight lie" occurs when a golfer's ball rests in an area with minimal grass beneath it. This sparse turf can complicate shots for amateur players, who often prefer having some grass cushioning under their ball for better contact.

**Toe**: The toe of a golf club refers to the area of the club face that is located beyond the grooves and is farthest from the golfer when addressing the ball. This part of the club is critical for understanding how different impacts can affect ball flight. In contrast, the opposite end of the club face is known as the "heel," which is closer to the golfer.

**Topped Shot**: A topped shot occurs when a golfer strikes the top half of the ball with the bottom edge of the club. This mis-hit results in a shot that typically travels only a short distance, often just a few yards, and can be quite frustrating for players as it fails to achieve intended distance or accuracy.

**Trail Foot or Hand**: The term "trail foot" or "trail hand" refers to the part of a golfer's body that is farthest from the target during their setup position when preparing to hit the ball. For right-handed golfers, this would be their right foot and right hand, while for left-handed golfers, it would be their left foot and left hand. Understanding this positioning is essential for proper swing mechanics.

**Triple Bogey**: A triple bogey, commonly referred to as a "trip," occurs when a golfer completes a hole with a score that is three strokes over par. For example, if a hole has a par of 4, scoring 7 on that hole would result in a triple bogey. This term reflects performance relative to par and can impact overall scoring in a round.

**Unplayable Lie**: An unplayable lie refers to a situation where a golfer's ball is in play but positioned in such a way that making an effective swing or advancing it becomes impossible. In such cases, golfers have the option to declare their ball unplayable according to the Rules of Golf. Once declared unplayable, there are three relief options available, all requiring taking one penalty stroke before proceeding with play.

**Up:** In match play, a player who has won more holes than they have lost is considered to be "up" in the match. For instance, if a player has won five holes and lost four, that player is "one up."

**Up and Down:** This term refers to a situation where a player does not reach the green in regulation (which is two strokes under par for that hole) but successfully pitches the ball onto the green and then holes it in one additional stroke.

**Uphill Lie:** An uphill lie occurs when a player's ball rests on an uneven surface, specifically when their front foot is positioned higher than their back foot due to the slope of the ground.

**USGA:** The acronym stands for the United States Golf Association, which serves as the governing body for golf in both the United States and Mexico. The USGA oversees the national handicap system and is responsible for producing and interpreting the Rules of Golf.

**USGTF:** The acronym stands for the United States Golf Teachers Federation, which is recognized as the largest organization globally dedicated to the intensive training and certification of elite golfers. Its primary mission is to prepare individuals to teach and coach golfers across all levels of skill, age, gender, and ethnicity. Upon successful completion of its courses, the USGTF awards a diploma of certification. To maintain this certification, members must remain in good standing within the organization.

**Vardon Grip**: This grip style is named after Harry Vardon, a renowned British golfer active during the late 19th and early 20th centuries. Vardon was instrumental in popularizing this particular grip technique, which is commonly known today as the "overlapping" grip. This method involves overlapping the little finger of the trailing hand over the index finger of the leading hand, providing stability and control during a golf swing.

**Waggle**: A waggle refers to a small movement that golfers perform to help alleviate tension before addressing the ball. Typically, this motion consists of one to three gentle waggles that serve as a way for players to relax and focus before executing their shot.

**Winter Rules**: This term describes a local rule that allows players to improve their lie within designated areas due to adverse course conditions typically associated with winter weather. Under winter rules, golfers may be permitted to clean or move their ball in order to ensure fair play despite challenging conditions on the course.

**Watery Grave:** This term refers to a situation in golf where a player hits their ball into a body of water, such as a pond or lake. The phrase likens the water to a grave, suggesting that the ball has found its final resting place there.

**Weak Grip:** A weak grip in golf is characterized by the positioning of the hands on the club such that the 'V' shapes formed between the thumbs and forefingers point towards the left shoulder (for right-handed golfers). This grip can lead to undesirable outcomes, particularly for amateur players, often resulting in a slice—a shot that curve dramatically to the right.

**Whiff:** In golfing terminology, a "whiff" occurs when a golfer attempts to strike the ball but completely misses it. This can happen due to poor timing or misjudgment during the swing.

**Wood:** The term "wood" refers to any golf club that traditionally had a wooden head. In modern times, however, these clubs are typically constructed from metal composites. Woods are designed for long-distance shots and are generally used for teeing off or hitting from fairways.

**Worm Burner:** A "worm burner" is slang for a poorly executed shot where the ball either barely lifts off the ground or remains entirely on

The Journey Begins

the ground after being struck. This type of shot is often unintentional and indicates an error in technique.

**X-outs:** These are golf balls that are typically sold at a reduced price due to minor cosmetic imperfections that occur during the manufacturing process.

**Yank:** This term describes a golf shot that veers offline to the left, commonly referred to as a "pull."

**Yardage:** This term indicates the distance between the golfer's ball and their intended target.

**Yips:** The yips are a frustrating condition in golf characterized by involuntary muscle spasms or mental blocks that disrupt a golfer's ability to execute fundamental tasks. This issue primarily affects putting, leading to erratic swing motions that can negatively impact the shot.

**Zip:** This term refers to the backspin applied to the golf ball upon impact, which causes it to stop quickly when it lands on the green or, in some cases, even roll backward.

# Epilogue:
# Your Journey Begins

As we reach the end of this guide, remember that golf is more than just a sport—it's a lifelong journey of growth, challenge, and joy. Whether you're picking up a club for the first time or seeking to refine your skills, the path ahead is filled with opportunities for both personal and athletic development.

Throughout this book, we've covered everything from the fundamental grip to advanced course management strategies. But perhaps the most important lesson is this: every golfer's journey is unique. There will be triumphant birdies and frustrating bogeys, perfect drives and wayward approaches. These experiences aren't just part of the game—they're what make golf such a compelling pursuit.

Remember that the greatest golfers in history once stood where you stand now. They learned the same basic grips, struggled with similar swing mechanics, and faced the same mental challenges. What set them apart wasn't innate talent alone, but their dedication to improvement and their love for the game.

As you step onto the course, carry with you not just the technical knowledge from these pages, but also the spirit of golf—its traditions, etiquette, and the camaraderie it fosters. Use the strategies and tips provided here as your foundation, but don't be afraid to develop your own style and approach to the game.

Golf will challenge you physically and mentally. It will test your patience and resolve. But it will also reward you with moments of pure joy, lasting friendships, and the satisfaction of personal achievement. Whether you're aiming to compete at a high level or simply enjoy weekend rounds with friends, the journey ahead is yours to shape.

So grab your clubs, step onto the tee, and begin your adventure in this magnificent game. Remember: every great golfer started with a single swing.

Welcome to the wonderful world of golf. Your journey begins now.

Glen Bowen
USGTF Certified Professional Golf Coach

# About the Author

## Certified Golf Professional and Inventor

Glen Bowen is a Certified Professional Golf Coach, affiliated with the United States Golf Teachers Federation (USGTF) and the United States Golf Association (USGA). With over two decades of experience, he provides personalized golf instruction in Salado, (Central) Texas.

Bowen is inventor of the Firecracker® golf tee, which was awarded "Best in Class" by Golf Test USA in competition with other leading tees and is approved by the USGA for tournament play.

He served as a medic in the U.S. Air Force during the Vietnam War and later was bestowed with an honorary commission as Admiral in the Texas Navy by Governor Rick Perry for his contributions to Texas.

www.ingramcontent.com/pod-product-compliance
Lightning Source LLC
Chambersburg PA
CBHW042315120626
46547CB00022B/2109